CHOKED PIPES

Reforming Pakistan's Mixed Health System

CHOKED PIPES

Reforming Pakistan's Mixed Health System

SANIA NISHTAR

Foreword by

JULIO FRENK

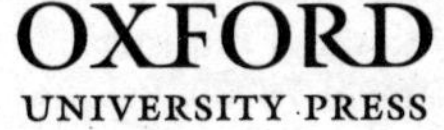

OXFORD
UNIVERSITY PRESS

Great Clarendon Street, Oxford OX2 6DP

Oxford University Press is a department of the University of Oxford.
It furthers the University's objective of excellence in research, scholarship,
and education by publishing worldwide in

Oxford New York

Auckland Cape Town Dar es Salaam Hong Kong Karachi
Kuala Lumpur Madrid Melbourne Mexico City Nairobi
New Delhi Shanghai Taipei Toronto

with offices in

Argentina Austria Brazil Chile Czech Republic France Greece
Guatemala Hungary Italy Japan Poland Portugal Singapore
South Korea Switzerland Turkey Ukraine Vietnam

Oxford is a registered trade mark of Oxford University Press
in the UK and in certain other countries

First published 2010

ISBN 978-0-19-547969-0

Typeset in Minion Pro
Printed in Pakistan by
Kagzi Printers, Karachi.
Published by
Ameena Saiyid, Oxford University Press
No. 38, Sector 15, Korangi Industrial Area, PO Box 8214
Karachi-74900, Pakistan.

Dedication

Dedicated to the silent and unjustified suffering of millions of individuals for whom the right to health remains unrealized—and whose lives I strive and aspire to touch

Contents

Foreword

In the past few years, health has increasingly been recognized as a key component of global security, sustainable economic growth, and good governance. As a result of this consensus, its importance in the global agenda has escalated, leading to unprecedented growth in development assistance for health.[1]

Such support for health is more than welcome. However, it is essential to recognize that this is a necessary but not sufficient condition. Meeting the health challenges of today's changing world requires more money for health, as well as development of the capacity to deliver—in the words of the legendary Professor Ramalingaswami: 'more health for the money.' So although resources are still short of need, it has been realized that additional funding will only be available if national and local health systems are strengthened. The focus is increasingly shifting towards accountability for results. In a virtuous circle, those results will be crucial for maintaining the momentum of increased funding for health.

The growing realization of the importance of health systems is reflected in the set of bilateral and multilateral initiatives, which have come forth during the past two years, to strengthen this area of work. It is interesting to notice that some of these initiatives are being promoted by actors, not traditionally involved in health matters, such as the G8 and the office of the Secretary General of the United Nations. This broad interest reflects the fact that health is being recognized, not only as a specific sector under the responsibility of specialized ministries of health and international agencies, but also as a social objective, with deep implications for every other area of human endeavour. Alongside its technical dimensions, health has profound economic, political, and ethical dimensions. As a universally shared value, health is an indicator of the general progress of a society and a reflection of its success in securing equal opportunities for all its members. Because of these broader implications, health indicators are a key component of the Human Development Index and health targets figure prominently in the Millennium Development Goals (MDGs).

This recent concern for health systems is also the expression of an effort to balance the excessive emphasis that global health initiatives had placed on vertical programmes devoted to control specific diseases. We are in need of 'magic bullets,' it is true, but we also need 'magic guns,'[2] and those guns are health systems. Unfortunately, there is still not a clear idea of what health systems should do and accomplish. It is, therefore, essential to improve understanding of this crucial component of every society.

The main virtue of *Choked Pipes: Reforming Pakistan's Mixed Health System* lies in its clear understanding of the boundaries, purposes, and functions of health systems. This provides a coherent framework for discussing the evolution of the Pakistani health system since its inception, its previous reform efforts, and its present configuration, as well as for presenting a comprehensive reform agenda.

Sania Nishtar recognizes that the health status of a population is dependent on a broad set of variables, many of which are modifiable only through inter-sectoral policies. For this reason, she constantly discusses the global and national context in which social and health policies in Pakistan have been implemented. In fact, the final part of the book divides the discussion of the reform agenda into two sections: reform outside of the healthcare system and reform within the healthcare system. However, in the presentation of what she calls the definitional context of the book, she also acknowledges that health systems have an important bearing on the health conditions of individuals and populations and that efforts should be made to improve their performance. In this process, she adopts a WHO definition of health system that relates it to the production of actions whose primary purpose is to improve or maintain health.[3]

The richest part of this book is devoted to description of the main functions developed within Pakistan's health system. This description, which excels for its clear order and thoroughness, offers a great variety of clues to the poor performance of health services in Pakistan. Part II opens with an explicit attempt to clarify what I have called the 'black box' and the 'black hole' misconceptions about health systems.[4] With this purpose in mind, Nishtar describes in detail, the key functions of a health system as applied to the Pakistani case: stewardship or governance, mobilization of financial resources, service delivery, and resource generation (including the development and distribution of human resource, drugs, technologies, and information systems).

In relation to governance, one of the salient features of Nishtar's analysis is the importance given both to the design as well as the implementation of strategic policies, regulations, and inter-sectoral coordination, and to the exercise of power by a great variety of political actors, including state actors, private providers, beneficiaries, NGOs, academic institutions, think tanks, and the media, amongst others. Ministries of health would be unable to articulate inter-sectoral interventions that affect the social determinants of health in the absence of a broad regulatory and convening capacity to promote health policies, including safety measures to prevent traffic accidents, norms to promote occupational health, and taxes to combat tobacco consumption. The attention to the distribution and use of power is equally important. Nishtar correctly argues that a reform is a profoundly political process. In this regard, she goes as far as to state that the main impediment to a broad reform process in the health sector of Pakistan has been 'the country's political, law and order, and geostrategic situation, which has overwhelmed the state apparatus and has crowded out the space for structural changes.'

Regarding the financing function, the most relevant feature of the Pakistani health system, as in many low and middle income countries, is the predominance of private expenditure, more specifically of out-of-pocket payments, a risk which households are exposed to incurring in health shocks. Nishtar explores the possibility of expanding the pooling base through various mechanisms, both in the formal as well as the informal sectors of the economy in order to improve the sufficiency and fairness of health financing in Pakistan. She recognizes that a social insurance model is not feasible there, since the country 'neither has the potential to generate enough revenue in the short term, nor can it generate the needed level of resources from payroll taxes because a majority of its workforce is employed in the informal sector.' For this reason, she discusses the potential of social protection schemes and community health insurance.

The main challenge in the delivery of health services in Pakistan is the expansion of coverage. In this regard, Nishtar proposes the definition of a package of essential services strongly associated to the MDGs, to which everybody should have access. To expand the supply of basic care, she suggests contracting non-state providers of primary health care services.

Two other major challenges in this domain are quality assurance and malpractices including staff absenteeism, dual job-holding, and theft of supplies. These practices are common both in the public as well as private health care delivery sectors and should immediately be addressed if the credibility of a reform effort is to be guaranteed.

In the resource generation domain, the most pressing problem, as in most health systems in developing nations, is related to the availability of human resource. In Pakistan, there is a reasonable supply of doctors but a shortage of nurses, dentists, midwives, and other health personnel. There is also a generalized problem of distribution due to several factors including lack of incentives and poor public infrastructures in rural and suburban areas. These factors drive providers to large towns, big facilities, and the private sector. In addition, there is a problem of capacities, which needs to be addressed through the strengthening of undergraduate and postgraduate education, in-service training, and continuing medical education. A key component of this effort should be directed towards addressing the serious shortage of health care managers, which limits the viability of any institutional reform.

Nishtar also acknowledges that no health system can succeed if providers lack the basic inputs for provision of care. Most of the recent increases in development cooperation for health have been directed to expanding the supply of drugs, vaccines, bed nets, and other technologies. However, these technologies must be embedded in a set of systems or sub-systems (procurement, information, personnel, etc.) designed to ensure the timely conjunction of human, financial, technological, and knowledge resources. One very positive aspect of the recent global initiatives on health systems strengthening is that they address many of these crucial issues.

Finally, Pakistan should also make an effort to build strong institutions. Nishtar's concern for this component is made evident when she concludes that 'the most important impediment to reform in Pakistan is the country's public sector institutional culture, which is focused on short-term goals as opposed to evidence-based, long-term enduring actions with potential to bring sustainable change.'

The book ends with a brilliant defence of a realistic but ambitious health reform agenda for Pakistan. It is realistic as it underscores the need for what Nishtar calls a 'multi-stakeholder sign-up to a *Reform Agenda* and a phased approach.' It is ambitious as it calls for the creation of major fiscal space to finance an effort that seeks to reform all basic functions of the health system in order to improve the health conditions of the Pakistani population.

Choked Pipes: Reforming Pakistan's Mixed Health System shows that the dilemma between local and global research is a false one. Globalization can turn conceptual frameworks, analytical methods, and policy experiences into international public goods. These goods can then be brought to the domestic policy agenda to address local problems, as illustrated by this outstanding discussion of the performance of Pakistan's health system and its potential for reform. The circle is brilliantly closed by the many lessons that this book brings to the shared search for better health systems throughout the world.

Julio Frenk
Dean
Harvard School of Public Health

Preface

I have worked on this publication with a conscious effort to serve two objectives. On the one hand, I have presented my viewpoint on reforming Pakistan's health system, and whilst doing so, have highlighted the salience of systemic impediments, which hinder efforts aimed at development in general. By drawing an analogy to a 'choked pipe,' the title of this publication underscores a key point—systems plagued by systemic challenges simply cannot deliver on desired public policy endpoints. Understanding these challenges and the means of their mitigation assume great importance in Pakistan at a time when the need to deliver welfare has never been more dire, given the country's prevailing geopolitical challenges.

Secondly, I have attempted to frame the discussion so that Pakistan's example can be of relevance to other developing countries as well. Health systems issues are unique to countries and are deeply interwoven with their body politic—so are the solutions. The US connotation and context of health reform—a subject of contemporary relevance—for example, has very little bearing on reform models elsewhere. That notwithstanding, there are reasons why the Mixed Health Systems Syndrome and its determinants and manifestations described in the context of Pakistan hold relevance for other developing countries, as has been described.

In presenting a viewpoint on directions for reform, I have emphasized the need for reform in key areas relevant to governance at the broader state level as being critical to the success of reform within the health system. With reference to the latter, I have articulated a set of synchronized policy, legislative, and institutional measures, which can be implemented in a phased manner. In doing so, an attempt has been made to draw on existing opportunities in the country. Pakistan's extensive private sector and the opportunities that exist to exercise leverage on the potential within public-private engagement to make pluralism in service delivery work for equity and quality, is one of them. The promising prospects of harnessing the potential within the country's telecommunication boom to mainstream technology in health systems for gains at several levels, is another. In the third place stands the potential within Pakistan's extensive institutional structure, which can be reformed through regulatory interventions and incentive and payment systems so that various factions can be empowered with respect to stewardship, implementation, and regulatory arrangements.

I have also commented on ongoing initiatives within the broader sphere of state governance to show how these can impact the right to health, health status, and health systems performance. A number of discussions in various sections of this publication are relevant in this regard. Notable amongst these is the discussion on socio-economic rights in view of the ongoing parliamentary deliberations on constitutional amendments; the section on decentralization in view of the present uncertain fate of the local government system; and the discussion around transparency-promoting reform with reference to the currently growing interest in this area.

I have invested time to conceptualize and articulate this reform agenda with the hope that the state will develop its capacity to strengthen its 'systems pipes,' which can then serve as a vehicle, not only for delivering healthcare but also for streamlining other conduits for targeting welfare to the people of Pakistan—a critical prerequisite for human security.

Sania Nishtar
Islamabad
October 4, 2009

Précis

This book presents the author's perspective on reforming Pakistan's health system—a system that is known to have underperformed over the last six decades. The analysis and directions for reform proposed herein also have a bearing on health systems in other developing countries. Additionally, they are relevant to current efforts aimed at achieving global development goals in today's macroeconomically constrained environment and meeting broader development objectives in the context of Pakistan's prevailing geostrategic challenges. The importance and relevance of a discussion on health reform in a given developing country with broader global and national development objectives has been underscored in three areas.

First and foremost, stand the global and domestic fiscal space constraints—an environment in which downsizing of public financing for health is feared, at a time when evidence from half-way mark reviews on progress towards meeting the Millennium Development Goals (MDGs), is calling for efforts to scale up funding.[5] While governments and international agencies strive to secure resources for development in this milieu, they are also focusing attention on ways to improve returns on spending by seeking to address constraints imposed by poorly functioning public systems. Limited understanding of the levers of change that can improve systems functioning in resource-challenged settings is an impediment in this regard. By illustrating the determinants of poor health systems performance in Pakistan's context, this book is a step towards bringing clarity in that direction—Pakistan's example can be of relevance to health and social sector systems in many other developing countries.

Secondly, this book has been compiled at a critical time in the evolution of interest in health systems in global health. Decades of disease-specific focus within the context of earlier efforts aimed at infectious disease control and later, the HIV and AIDS epidemic and the MDGs have brought to attention the inability of weak health systems to deliver on disease-specific targets and have exposed structural weaknesses in health systems. This realization is marked by the beginning of a shift in global health from *diseases* to *systems*.[6] The new emphasis on health systems creates an imperative for developing normative guidance to strengthen health systems around the world—an increasingly challenging goal, given the diversity in health systems designs. Notwithstanding many differences, healthcare in a majority of the low- and middle-income countries is delivered by what can be described as a *Mixed Health System*—a health system in which out-of-pocket payments and market provision of services predominates as a means of financing and providing services in an environment where publicly-funded government health delivery coexists with privately-financed market delivery.[7]

The public market interaction and its manifestations, evidenced by compromised equity and quality in healthcare delivery can be described as the *Mixed Health Systems Syndrome*—the denotation of syndrome refers to a set of concurrently appearing characteristics, which indicate poor performance with respect to key indicators of health systems performance. Although this book describes this interaction in Pakistan's environment, the discussion and its context is relevant to many developing countries. By developing normative guidance to mainstream equity and quality in Pakistan's Mixed Health System, this book attempts to make an initial contribution to this least developed area in global health—as Pakistan's Mixed Health System can be regarded as a developing country prototype, generic elements from this normative framework can also be helpful for other developing countries. A discussion on equity in the space of a Mixed Health System can also be leveraged to galvanize a shift towards a just social order and universal coverage in health, in the broader context of the imperative created by the recent financial crisis to foster a greater oversight role of the state over markets.

Thirdly, Pakistan stands as a country where the need to remedy welfare and social sector systems—of which health is most important—has become an urgent priority for reasons beyond the idealistic resolve to achieve egalitarian objectives. In the midst of many threats *by* and *to* a society deeply divided on religious and ethnic grounds, the delivery of equitable welfare services is the only tool to protect the rapidly burgeoning and impoverished base of the population pyramid from being exploited by extremist elements. However, targeting of social services, which appears a straightforward objective in many other parts of the world if resources are available, is becoming an exceedingly complex and impossible task to achieve in Pakistan's environment, given the skew in certain fundamentals of governance, resulting from weaknesses in the political process and the means of targeting services. This book has attempted to address the core determinants of these failures by working backwards along the causal chain to identify the evolution of causes. In doing so, the book describes the *Triad of Determinants* that lead to mayhem in the Mixed Health System—low public funding for health, a poorly-regulated private sector and differences in incentives as a result thereof, and lack of transparency in governance. The resulting complex interaction undermines the equity and quality objectives of the health system through many pathways. This triad holds true for most social sectors in addition to health, not just in Pakistan, but also in many other developing countries.

The publication sets out by following the history of health restructuring and 'reform' attempts over the last 62 years of the country's existence. The account draws attention to the plethora of initiatives and the lack of a sustained approach to reform. Many post-colonial nation-states will identify themselves with these 'reform' attempts given the common multilateral frameworks from which they emanate. The account, in addition to a description of Pakistan's health systems, constitutes Part I of this book. The latter also explains how mutually exclusive vertical systems can exist in their own right within a country setting—another description, which can be contextualized to many other countries. Part II presents an analysis of issues within individual health system streams. In addition to the World Health Organization's (WHO) six health systems domains—service delivery, health workforce, information, financing, governance, and medicines and related products[8]—this publication frames technology as an additional input-level domain, on the premise that its potential to enhance efficiency and connectivity, and control errors and costs would bring value to a resource-constrained developing country.

The evidence presented in this book draws on findings from research conducted by the author over the last two years. Mixed methods—qualitative and quantitative research—were employed for the analyses. These included a review of academic and grey literature, semi-structured interviews, focus group discussions with key informants, expert consultations and a series of online surveys. Methodological details are forthcoming in a set of scientific papers.

The analysis illustrates a number of institutionalized challenges in each health systems domain. Each of the respective chapters in Part II maps the cycle of challenges and elaborates on how these are exacerbated by poorly performing governance and accountability arrangements. Although the interaction has been described for the health sector, the dynamics hold true for most other social sectors as well. Understanding the dynamics of these impediments is critical at a time when the need to target welfare to the people of Pakistan has never been more urgent, not just as a domestic goal but also as an international target. The brief summary articulating the directions for reform at the conclusion of each of the chapters in Part II is supplemented by a stand-alone section on *Health Reform* as Part III of this book, which outlines the envisaged directions of policy, institutional, and legislative restructuring. It has also been outlined in a *Scaffold for Health Policy*—another output of the author's contribution to assist with health reform in Pakistan[9]—as an Appendix.

In sum, the book's *Reform Agenda* outlines four areas for reform both within as well as outside of the healthcare system. Broader systems constraints within the remit of the political economy is the first area. The Reform Agenda underscores the need to focus on debt limitation, fiscal responsibility, measures to broaden the tax base, pro-poor growth, and overall transparency and effectiveness in governance, as these are deemed critical for improving health status and health systems performance. Secondly, it lays emphasis on increasing the base of public sources of financing for health and management reengineering of public service delivery. The former includes incremental increases in revenues to support essential services, broadening the base of social protection for the informally employed sector, and maximizing pooling through insurance for the formally employed sector. It is envisaged that with adequate resourcing and management reengineering, workforce can be retained in the public sector, availability of medicines, supplies and infrastructure can be improved, and public facilities can be better managed.

In the third place, the Reform Agenda calls for market harnessing regulatory approaches in order to broaden the first point of contact in Primary Health Care as well as enable purchase of services in order to achieve equitable access to care. The fourth area is institutional reform of state agencies mandated in a health role in order to enhance their normative and oversight capacity to oversee provision of services, ideally with institutional separation of policy-making, and implementing and regulatory functions. Lastly, the Reform Agenda calls for some additional measures. Notable amongst these are the use of technology in order to assist with securing the distribution chain, making procurements transparent, optimizing time and connectivity in health information systems, and bridging gaps in training, continuing education, and information dissemination.

The Reform Agenda envisages implementing these changes in a step-wise manner. Step I focuses on developing a national consensus on the reform agenda and increasing public financing for health. Step II involves bracing the health information system and pulling a thread through existing evidence. Step III has three components—strengthening institutions; honing norms, and mainstreaming technology. Step IV is focused on prototyping alternative service delivery and financing mechanisms whereas Step V is centred on scaling up. Ongoing generation of evidence and its mainstreaming into planning is deemed necessary for implementing this agenda.

Implementation of the multidimensional nature of reform proposed in this book necessitates political will, perseverance, consistency of policy direction over time, and the resolve and capacity to cascade multidimensional changes in a sequenced manner as tangible action into policies, laws, and institutional arrangements. The current political climate and institutional culture, which is marked by limited capacity, lack of transparency, and short-term orientation, creates an impediment to institutionalization of the substantive changes proposed herein. It is hoped that this effort, which is aimed at articulating a vision for health reform, will serve as a catalyst and lend impetus to positive change in Pakistan's institutional culture in the health sector. It is additionally envisaged that the normative parameters of relevance to mainstreaming equity in the Mixed Health System will be regarded as a useful contribution within the space of global health.

PART I

Pakistan's Health System

The first section of this book presents an overview of efforts made in the last 62 years to reform Pakistan's health system and attempts to highlight weaknesses of approaches adopted in the past. It also outlines the existing configuration of the country's health systems and presents a brief overview of the factors responsible for poor health status.

Chapter 1

Health Systems Reform: A Historical Perspective

1.1 Health as a human right

The ultimate objective of health reform is to secure better health outcomes. The discussion around health reform, therefore, becomes inextricably linked to the issue of socio-economic rights, the matter of their enforcement, and the challenges in realizing the right to health. In many ways, healthcare reform conceptually represents the 'battle of socio-economic rights.' If health is regarded as a fundamental human right and if the right to health is enforceable, then there can be a much stronger case for necessary investments to support healthcare reform. A country's constitutional position on socio-economic rights and the manner in which they can be enforced, therefore, assume great importance in the entire discussion on health reform and can, at least in theory, lend impetus to generating political will and the necessary resources to support reform.

The Universal Declaration of Human Rights (UDHR) forms the basis of understanding the concept of socio-economic rights and the question of their enforcement. The UDHR was initially intended as one instrument but was later bifurcated into two distinct and different covenants, namely the International Covenant on Civil and Political Rights (ICCPR) and the International Covenant on Economic, Social, and Cultural Rights (ICESCR). Many states, which supported the separation, were of the opinion that the two sets of rights could not be equated and that social and economic prerogatives of citizens could not be the basis of binding obligations, in the way that civil and political rights needed to be. The split allowed states to adopt some rights and derogate others. However, despite the fact that more than 70 per cent of all nations have ratified the 1966 ICESCR, which makes the right to health an international obligation and despite WHO's declaration, which states that 'enjoyment of the highest attainable standard of health is one of the fundamental rights of every human being,' the reality is that the right to health has been neglected and violated in many parts of the world.

Recently, however, there has been a burgeoning international trend towards progressive interpretation of rights. Currently, there are 115 countries in the world, which recognize the constitutional right to health. Chile provided the first constitutional recognition in 1925. Over the last two decades, many Latin American courts, from both civil as well as common law jurisdictions, have handed down landmark decisions guaranteeing access to treatment affecting thousands of individuals. The movement for judicialization of health rights has largely been fuelled by challenges that states face to provide antiretroviral treatment and the treatment of other diseases, which cause catastrophic expenditure. Patients across Brazil, for example, have been turning to courts in recent years to access prescribed drugs ever since the 1996 legislation, which granted universal access to antiretroviral treatment. Since then, lawsuits all over the country have secured access to treatment for thousands of people.[10] In South Africa, ever since the constitution came into force in 1994, health rights together with housing rights have become the most important socio-economic rights cases considered by courts. In addition to individual treatment, public interest litigation cases affecting the right to health have also been those concerning protection of the environment, particularly in judgments from South Asian courts.[11]

This recent international trend towards progressive interpretation of rights and some recent normative frameworks, such as the adoption of a landmark resolution by the United Nations Human Rights Council, acknowledging preventable maternal mortality as a human rights issue,[12] represent a change from the previous discussions and connotations of reform, which centred on efficiency gains, as is described later in this chapter. The emerging paradigm shift can assume importance in shaping public policy in the context of the recent meltdown of the market and the consequent emergence of a new world order. The latter has created an imperative for national governments to exercise a stronger normative, regulatory, and oversight role and strengthen welfare systems. It is hoped that these recent developments will galvanize stronger national commitment for health across the developing world—a key prerequisite for reform. However, it must be appreciated that lack of constitutional recognition of the right to health is not necessarily a bar to consideration and enforcement, as in the case of the United Kingdom and Canada, where health is almost treated as a human right.

Under the Constitution of the Islamic Republic of Pakistan, most of the fundamental rights listed in Chapter 1, Part II—entitled Fundamental Rights—fall within the domain of civil and political rights. Socio-economic rights, including the rights to health and education, have not been explicitly recognized as rights in this chapter. However, a reference to socio-economic 'rights' features in two areas in the constitution. The Objectives Resolution, which forms the preamble to the constitution and was originally passed in 1946, makes an explicit reference to social justice as one of the five principles guiding the democratic state. Secondly, Article 25 and 38(d) of Chapter 2, Part II—entitled Principles of Policy—refers to 'Equality of citizens' and 'Promotion of social and economic well-being of the people', respectively. Other articles of relevance to health include Article 9 on 'Security of a person' and Article 14 on 'Inviolability of the dignity of man.'

Conventionally, these covenants are referred to as being the basis of the rights-based approach to health in Pakistan, with Article 8 and 9 read with Article 199 providing the basis for enforcement of fundamental rights. Article 9, in particular, has been broadly interpreted in case law in this regard. In addition, the government of Pakistan is also a signatory to a number of international commitments, which set out in detail, actions and mechanisms towards the rights-based approach to health—in particular, the Convention on the Rights of the Child,[13] the Convention on the Elimination of All Forms of Discrimination against Women,[14] the Declaration of Alma Ata,[15] the Programme of Action of the International Conference on Population and Development,[16] and the Beijing Platform for Action.[17] Unlike 115 countries of the world, Pakistan's constitution does not, however, explicitly recognize the right to health. The Objectives Resolution and the Principles of Policy cannot be directly enforced through courts. Despite these constraints, however, courts in Pakistan have previously handed down progressive decisions in public interest. These stem from the fact that the constitution regards life as a basic human right but does not define life. Over the years, a series of court judgments have taken a progressive interpretation of the word 'life' and have held that since the word has not been defined in the constitution, it does not have to be restricted to mere existence in contradistinction to death but should include within its ambit, any hazard to life, including ill health, both in individual as well as in communal settings.[18,19] In these cases, the court achieved equivalence between civil and political rights and their social and economic counterparts through the application of an expansive definition of right to life.

As this publication went to print, a Special Committee on Constitutional Reform is debating the construct of the 18th Amendment to the Constitution of Pakistan. Ideas are being mooted to holistically revisit the constitution this time round, as opposed to earlier amendments, which primarily focused on the power nexus. Within this context, calls to action have been drawing attention to the need for addressing the lack of clarity in relation to socio-economic rights.[20] If Pakistan explicitly recognizes the right to health, the case for health reform and the directions focused on universal coverage can become much stronger. Everyone deserves to have the basic requirements of health—both healthcare as well as the underlying determinants of health—proper nutrition, adequate sanitation, safe drinking water and environmental and occupational health.[21] The Reform Agenda articulated herein is grounded in the rights-based approach to health, recognizing health as a basic development need.

1.2 Lessons from around the world: A snapshot

Healthcare reform has a different connotation in different settings. Health reform, which denotes positive change,[22] or more explicitly, sustained, purposeful, and fundamental change,[23] is an umbrella term used for major changes in health policy or in the public policy sphere that impact health and/or healthcare. The configuration of health reform is usually unique to a specific health systems setting. As such, therefore, reform represents great diversity in terms of the measures or the package of measures that can be introduced under its rubric. Over the years, countries have introduced health reform for achieving various end-points—efficiency gain, cost containment, managerial and institutional transformation, coverage and access enhancement, etc. In the United States, for example, where a publicly-funded system exists alongside a more predominant market system of pooling and provision, reform proposals have centred on removal of the private insurance market and establishment of a public option, premium subsidies to help individuals purchase health insurance, medical liability reform, policy options to reduce healthcare costs, and others to improve decision-making. The recent resounding enthusiasm for healthcare reform and divergent views about the type of fixes are drawing attention to some important questions that centre on issues of the right to healthcare, quality achieved for the sums spent, and sustainability of expenditures.[24]

In the welfare model of the United Kingdom, on the other hand, where a publicly funded National Health Service has gone through various stages of reform over the last six decades, elements of competition, patient choice, diversity of providers, freedom for hospitals, stronger commissioning, new payment mechanisms, and independent inspection of quality have strongly featured as elements of health reform. In both these developed nations, where there is a strong societal political culture and where healthcare often accounts for one of the largest areas of spending for both governments and individuals, health reform is surrounded by hotly-contested political debates and controversies. This is evidenced by the difference in opinion between the Conservative and the Labour Party over the introduction of the purchaser-provider split in the United Kingdom. The divergent views on the type of fixes currently being supported by the Democrats and the Republicans in the United States, with the former leaning towards broadening the base of insurance and the latter supporting open market competition in order to cut costs are also illustrative.

In Western Europe, evolutionary progress in the aftermath of the Second World War, led many countries towards comprehensive universal coverage, financed either by insurance or by revenues. Reforms in the health sector in some middle-income countries of Latin America and Eastern Europe, on the other hand, have largely been carried out by expanding medical insurance. In most of these cases, international financial organizations have assisted with reform. Cuba is perhaps the only country where reform was purely indigenous and was not supported by international agencies. It predated reform in other Latin American countries by two decades and was characterized by decentralization, emphasis on primary healthcare, and universal coverage.

The contemporary understanding of health reform in the developing countries in particular is shaped by reforms introduced by international agencies in the 1990s. These used a variety of entry points with organizational efficiency as an outcome—introducing insurance, changes in payment systems, decentralization, alternative modes of Primary Health Care (PHC) delivery, and hospital restructuring are examples of reform initiatives pursued by various countries in the past. Historically, health reform in many developing countries has previously been linked to the concept of neo-liberal reform. Overall, the latter promoted a package of measures, which included privatization of public enterprise, deregulation of the economy, liberalization of trade and industry, removal of controls on global financial flows, and reduction of public expenditures in many areas. Within this framework, healthcare reforms in most developing countries have previously sought to improve the efficiency and quality of Primary Health Care by structuring the role of the market in healthcare provision with separation of purchaser and provider functions as a major institutional overhaul. While some of these reform efforts have shown to influence access, quality, and efficiency,[25] these approaches have also raised many concerns and have come under criticism due to their perceived ideological conflict with the principles of Health for All.[26,27] It is important that in addition to efficiency gain, health reform should also be configured to impact outcomes, with fairness in financing, enhanced responsiveness, and reducing barriers to access as endpoints. Achieving these endpoints in the Mixed Health System necessitates restructuring both systems of health and governance. Strong political leadership, an astute implementation capacity, and people's participation are critical to the success of the needed transformational change.

The debate about the role of the state in health,[28,29] and the extent to which the private sector should be involved,[30,31] and regional examples,[32,33] indicate that any reform, as it attempts to harness the potential of the market, should not provide the state an opportunity to divest from one of its core responsibilities, which is to provide for the well-being of its citizens. The role of private provision can be important and public-private collaboration in health systems may be urgently needed but these must be fostered under the clear stewardship of the public sector.[34] The direction for reform of Pakistan's Mixed Health System articulated herein hinges on this principle. However, it is recognized that limited capacity and transparency within the state system would be key impediments in this connection and that measures need to be concomitantly taken to enhance these critical health systems functions.

The cases of Cuba, Kerala, and Costa Rica help to highlight the importance of public commitment to health.[35,36] In Cuba, health remains free, is accessible to everybody, and is relatively of good quality. There are some fundamental reasons for the success of the Cuban healthcare system. The socialist transformation of 1951 introduced elements that were particularly helpful for healthcare, their other gaps notwithstanding. Full commitment of the government in public policy terms to health and education and mass participation of the working class are amongst factors that have contributed to success. Today, Cuba's health indicators are comparable with countries such as the United States even though a huge difference exists in their respective levels of economic development and per capita income.[37] Other examples from around the world also show that where there is a sustained commitment by the government and where governments spend more relative to GDP on health, health outcomes are more desirable and are better distributed.[38]

Another example is that of Hong Kong, which has adopted healthcare financing and organizational health systems that are commonly seen in centrally planned economies while its economy functions as a highly capitalistic enterprise. This has enabled it to achieve health indicators comparable to the United States while spending 4.7 per cent of its GDP on health. China, on the other hand, spends 3.6 per cent of its GDP on health but has indicators comparable to many developing countries, largely as a result of integrating many features of healthcare systems associated with market economies while its overall economy is centrally planned.[39] More recent examples of progress in improving health indicators in Thailand,[40,41] Mexico,[42] and Tanzania,[43] also emphasize the importance of public commitment to health. Furthermore, it must be recognized that countries that have made progress in making structural changes at the PHC level—health systems reform has been most well-described at this level—through purchaser-provider separation and decentralization have been able to maximize efficiencies and broaden the outreach of service delivery through the commitment of governments that have the capacity to harness the strength of the market. Such models of service delivery reform, in isolation, are not a substitute for a government's commitment to health.[44,45]

Insights from these examples clearly indicate that as attempts are made to restructure healthcare systems, governments must not divest from one of their core public policy responsibilities, which is to ensure the well-being of its citizens. A commitment to health must be paralleled with support to other social sector areas as well so that the synergistic effect of improved education, gender equality, poverty alleviation, and increase in per capita income can interplay to improve health and other social outcomes in a holistic manner.

1.3 History of health reform in Pakistan

Various attempts have been made in the past to 'reform' the healthcare system in Pakistan. Efforts have emerged in many socio-political contexts, against the backdrop of various policy agendas and development strategies, varying economic opportunities, and the wave of globalization. Interplay of forces outside of the health sector has been critical in shaping developments relevant to health in Pakistan. As a result, a plethora of new initiatives and 'reforms' were introduced at various points in time by different governments (Figure 1). However, weaknesses in institutional capacity to sustain and support initiatives led to their discontinuation with changing governments or withdrawal of donor support. Most 'reforms' have remained poorly-evaluated and lessons learnt, if any, were seldom factored into planning.

The subsequent section of this chapter will provide a snapshot of reform-related initiatives in individual health systems domains. This is preceded by a historical account of health reform in the context of the history of development assistance received by Pakistan over the last 62 years.

1.3.1 Health reform and the history of development assistance

The history of health reform in Pakistan can best be tracked alongside a historical account of development assistance in the country. Understanding the historical perspective and dynamics of this relationship is important, as donors have had an important agenda-setting role in Pakistan with reference to health planning.

Several bilateral and multilateral development agencies, Global Health Initiatives (GHIs), private foundations, and other development

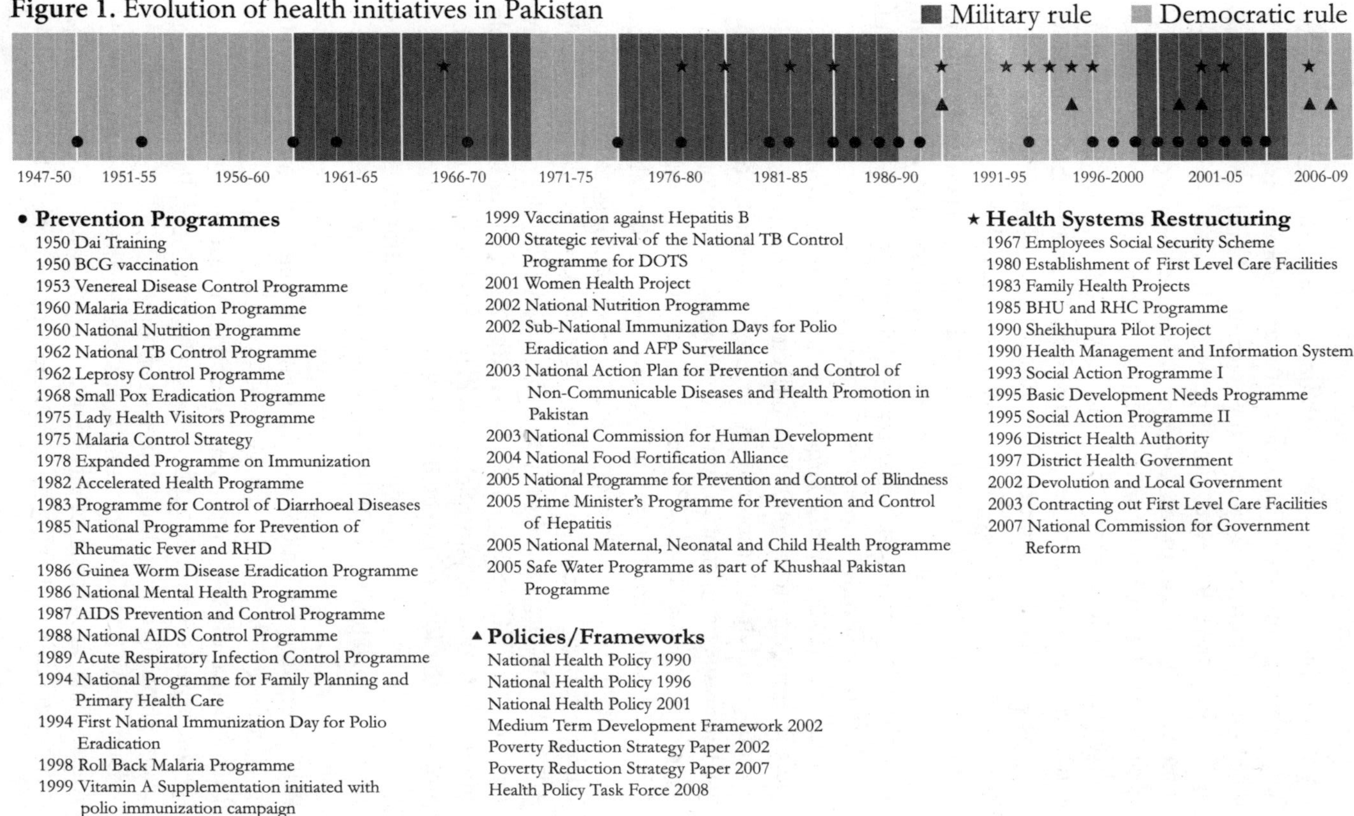

Figure 1. Evolution of health initiatives in Pakistan

windows are now part of the global health architecture, which plays an important role in financing and technically supporting health initiatives in developing countries. Since the 1940s, development assistance for the developing countries has undergone various stages of transition; trends in Pakistan have followed global patterns. In 1947—incidentally the same year that Pakistan was created—a large epidemiological outbreak of cholera in Egypt lent impetus to the development of tropical medicine for dealing with international outbreak containment in developing countries. Tropical medicine and tropical disease research, therefore, became a vehicle for channelling health-related development assistance to developing countries. Tropical disease research was an important source of capacity building in Pakistan as it supported doctoral training of many health professionals, who presently serve in key public health administrative roles within the country; however, many have also left for other opportunities, overseas.

Until the 1970s, WHO largely remained focused on the disease-specific approach to health. This reflected in Pakistan's public health planning, which correspondingly focused on small pox eradication, malaria eradication, control, and prevention; and control of a few other infectious diseases. In 1978, WHO launched the PHC movement at the Alma Ata Conference.[46] This shifted attention of the developing world to universal coverage and Health for All. As a response to this, Pakistan started establishing a large number of PHC facilities as a signatory to the Alma Ata Declaration. Shortly thereafter, however, the comprehensive approach to PHC envisaged by Alma Ata was perceived as non-viable, and in 1982, an alternative Selective PHC approach was launched. This promoted the idea of targeted interventions for childhood illnesses.[47] The UNICEF's Growth monitoring, Oral re-hydration, Breast-feeding and Immunization (GOBI) strategy against six vaccine preventable diseases, which selected four of the elements of PHC led the selective PHC campaign and subsequently UNICEF joined hands with WHO to introduce Integrated Management of Childhood Illnesses (IMCI). This selective disease-focused agenda, which was aimed at improving specific aspects of individual health, had its imprint on Pakistan's public health planning during the 1980s and beyond.

Due to WHO's resource constraints during the 1980s and 90s, the World Bank and some other financial institutions assumed a more preeminent role in shaping the health development agenda, particularly in the health systems stream, as part of the implementation of neo-liberal macroeconomic policies and structural adjustment programmes. During this phase, a number of Social Action Programme-led systems reform pilots, which aimed to address management inefficiencies at the PHC level were implemented by rapidly changing democratic governments in Pakistan. These attempts aimed to address management inefficiencies at the PHC level by attempting to mainstream the purchaser-provider split, decentralize service delivery arrangements, and promote efficient management of resources. Most of these health reform pilots could not have an impact because of a number of institutional and political considerations. Therefore, any potential benefit of these approaches, encompassed within the principles of decentralization, subsidiarity, and technical and allocative efficiency, could not be capitalized.

Up until the 1990s, low- and middle-income countries received development assistance either from multilateral agencies, largely as credits or through bilateral donors and private foundations as grants. In the early 1990s, a range of multi-stakeholder governance-characterized global public-private partnerships—contemporaneously referred to as Global Health Initiatives—started evolving.[48] Global Health Initiatives represented a radical shift away from the United Nations and multilateral and bilateral agency-dominated donor support to a broader-based mode of governing development assistance, with participation from representatives of the industry, northern and southern NGOs and in the case of the Global Fund to Fight AIDS, Tuberculosis and Malaria (GFATM), disease communities. Many GHIs, including the Global Alliance for Vaccines and Immunization (GAVI), GFATM, Stop TB and Roll Back Malaria (RBM) were introduced in Pakistan during this period and currently operate by financing and technically supporting the national public health programmes. Issues emerging as a result of vertical management of these programmes, which were recognized at an early stage of their establishment, prevail to date and have not been addressed adequately. This has been discussed further in the chapter on *Service Delivery*.

In 2000, the Millennium Development Goals (MDGs) were stipulated by the UNDP. These were endorsed by all member countries of the United Nations and further reinforced the vertical disease-focused nature of development assistance. The then military government of Pakistan attempted to align its health sector priorities to meet these time-bound and outcome-based objectives. In the aftermath of 9/11, fiscal space constraints eased in Pakistan as a result of a number of factors. Consequently, government allocations and development assistance for health increased. However, development assistance has never been close to the monetary target of 0.7 per cent of the GDP of developed countries—articulated as Goal 8 of the MDGs—and estimated need of 0.54 per cent.[49] Conversely, a greater proportion of aid has been channelled to security and war efforts particularly in the aftermath of 9/11. In 2006, a review of progress at mid-point showed that Pakistan is off-track in achieving the MDGs.[50] During this phase of relative increase in fiscal resources for health, the public health agenda was broadened to MDG+ with the inclusion of hepatitis,[51] blindness,[52] and prevention and control of non-communicable diseases in public health planning—the latter in a pilot design.[53] Health systems strengthening was meant to be an indirect beneficiary through allocations for a programme dedicated to maternal and child health—a programme, which continues to suffer from several challenges. However, as the National Health Policy enunciated in 2001 remained focused on disease control during this period, the needed systems transformation could not be effectively mainstreamed.

Over the last two decades, health has been capturing a bigger share of development assistance globally, although major financial constraints remain to be addressed. The sectoral composition of development assistance has also been changing. This has been most notable in the context of the AIDS epidemic and later the MDGs. The emergence of AIDS in particular transformed the way in which the world engaged with global health—with great political zeal and advocacy. However, this also reinforced the disease-specific focus in global health and led countries to allocate indigenous resources vertically. The emergence of UNAIDS and the President's Emergency Plan for AIDS Relief (PEPFAR) further reinforced disease-specific planning. Health financing patterns in Pakistan closely followed international trends. Although Pakistan was not a PEPFAR country,[54] funding for HIV and AIDS dominated domestic as well as development assistance allocations for health. As opposed to this, non-communicable diseases and injuries, which accounted for more than 50 per cent of the disease burden, were not prioritized in public health planning.

During this era of disease-specific focus, it was perceived all along that investments in high priority diseases could strengthen health systems through a knock-on effect, particularly in the areas of human resource and procurement. That clearly was not the case and as disease-specific programmes got well on their way to implementation, concerns related to the inability of weak health systems to deliver on programme targets became a predominant concern. As a result of this realization, a shift in global health from *diseases* to *health systems strengthening* now seems to be underway.

The World Health Organization commenced its efforts with publication of the World Health Report 2000,[55] and the Joint Learning Initiative (JLI) report,[56] and subsequently hosted a meeting on the Montreax Challenge.[57] More recently, the Director General's High Level Consultation,[58] the Global Synergies initiative,[59] the Bamako Ministerial Declaration,[60] publication of two landmark reports,[61,62] regional charters and pronouncements,[63,64] and the recent Venice Statement,[65,66] indicate the organization's growing interest in the area. Major GHIs such as GAVI and GFATM are also now capitalizing health systems strengthening as conditionality for funding.[67,68] The emergence of new GHIs—Health Metrics Network,[69] the Global Workforce Alliance,[70] and the International Health Partnership[71]—explicitly in the systems domains, an emphasis on aid effectiveness through the Paris Declaration on Aid Effectiveness and the Accra Agenda,[72,73] and higher priority accorded to health systems by private foundations,[74,75] and G8,[76,77] are also indicative of a swing in global health.

The emerging transformation in global health from *diseases* to *health systems* is yet to fully cascade into planning and implementation in Pakistan. However, interest has been sparked in the area with the publication of the Gateway Paper.[78,79] Its vision cascaded into Pakistan's Poverty Reduction Strategy Paper II.[80] The recent initiative of the government of Pakistan in the area of maternal and child health is also, to some extent, orientated towards health systems strengthening. Donors also appear to be taking a more proactive role in health systems strengthening, as is evidenced by the support lent by the Norway Pakistan Partnership Initiative (NPPI) to the maternal and child health programme in Sindh.

The afore-stated account has attempted to follow the evolution of development assistance in relation to the health sector, chronologically. Within this context, it is also important to recognize that because of many interventions, over time, the aid architecture has become increasingly complicated, with many agencies pursuing various objectives. A number of challenges have emerged as results of this. Over the years, donors have also rallied around a number of approaches and channels of disbursement and have experimented with project assistance, programme assistance and budget support. Strategies and instruments of donor disbursement have been described later in the chapter on *Health Financing*.

The recent global financial crisis was a watershed in global health, both in terms of its implications for development assistance as well as the imperatives it created for a just social order.[81] Pakistan is in a unique position in terms of development assistance, even during the financial crisis, as a result of recognition by donor countries of the need to resource welfare activities in the country in view of its geostrategic challenges—the US envisages channelling US $1.5 billion in bilateral development assistance annually, for the next five years.[82] However, it is hoped that alongside this, donor countries will also review their broader development footprint and in addition to committing traditional bilateral and multilateral assistance, will also assist in wiping out external indebtedness and mainstreaming a more conducive framework for trade—both these factors can have a more sustainable impact on development, welfare and Pakistan's proactive and peaceful role in a globalized world.

1.3.2 History of institutional reform

The section on the Ministry of Health in the chapter on *Institutional Reform* outlines roles of the Ministry of Health and the current weaknesses in capacities, which constrain its ability to perform those roles. Although efforts have been made from time to time, to bridge weaknesses, a consolidated plan to reform the ministry has not been tabled, to date. Therefore, the role of the Ministry of Health as an organizational entity constitutionally mandated to spearhead policy change has been unremarkable, over time. The Ministry of Health has limited institutional capacity for policy development and analysis. A National Health Policy Unit existed within the Ministry of Health for over 10 years but suffered from lack of ownership and remained poorly resourced. The unit has now been abolished and a health systems strengthening unit is in the process of being created in its place in order to comply with GAVI's new conditionality.[83] Additionally, there are no formal institutional linkages between the evidence-information-planning-policy cycle despite the existence of various streams of health information in the country.

During Pakistan's 62-year history, two health policies have been pronounced—in 1997 and 2001. Earlier in 1990, a draft health policy was tabled for Cabinet approval but could not be enunciated as a policy. Recently, efforts have been initialized to develop a new health policy.[84] Details have been discussed in the chapter on *Health Reform*.

There are limited examples of efforts that could have potentially led to institutional restructuring. At the provincial level, health regularity authorities were created in the North-West Frontier Province (NWFP) and Balochistan, but failed to serve their given mandate, as governments appeared reluctant to relinquish controls vested in departments and entrust independent regulatory functions to autonomous agencies. A Cabinet approval was granted to create a Drug Regulatory Authority in 2005. However, needed action to establish its structure has not been forthcoming. No serious effort has been made to separate policy-making, regulatory, and implementation functions within government agencies in the health sector or to grant attached agencies, the level of administrative and financial autonomy needed for appropriate functioning. In 2005, a National Commission was mandated with the overall task of reforming the executive branch of the government. After three years of analytical work, the commission's recommendations were published.[85] These recommendations were not implemented after change in government in 2008.

In comparison to the Ministry of Health, the provinces have been more proactive in attempting to restructure health systems. However, a downside of this relates to the lack of uniform understanding of the reform process across the country, as efforts at the provincial level have burgeoned in the absence of clear signalling of policy directions from the Ministry of Health. At the provincial level, NWFP and Punjab took a lead in experimenting with reform. In either case, development agencies actively supported reform initiatives.

The NWFP health reform programme has been supported by German bilateral assistance. The donor agency has played an advisory and technically supportive role in the areas of decentralization, health financing, quality, and human resource management in addition to institutionally supporting NWFP's Health Sector Reform Unit (HSRU).[86] The HSRU made a difference in terms of initializing hospital autonomy reform, assisting with legislative change in the area, and sparking political interest in social health insurance. However, HSRU has neither been able to mainstream a consolidated vision for reform in the province nor has it been able to streamline controversial initiatives such as institution-based private practice, which was initialized in 2001 and subsequently dismantled. The HSRU has also been unable to play a catalytic role in fully galvanizing NWFP's Health Regulatory Authority. The latter could have played an important role in restructuring service delivery arrangements.

The NWFP health reform programme has also received technical assistance from multilateral sources to plan for reform, conduct sector analyses, and strengthen institutional capacity.[87] Reports of sector analyses are not available in the public domain.[88] Health-related reforms in NWFP have also been part of broader human development reforms, which have supported specific activities such as supplementary immunization.[89] In addition, health should have also benefited from financial sector management reforms in the province.[90] The translation of fiscal support in these areas into tangible outcomes has not been evident.

Punjab has a long-standing history of experimenting with a range of health reform initiatives in the areas of institutional restructuring, PHC, and hospitals—in each case, official development agencies have actively supported reform. The contemporary institutional history of health reform dates back to the 1990s and has been described in the section on *Decentralization,* later in this chapter. Reform initiatives relevant to PHC and hospitals have also been discussed in respective sections. Non-governmental Organizations (NGOs) played a major role in institutionalizing reform of PHC in the province, as has been described in the section on *Service delivery at the primary healthcare level,* later in this chapter.

As the most populous province of the country, Punjab benefited the most from the increase in fiscal space in Pakistan post-9/11,2001 onwards. The Planning Commission, Punjab created strategic frameworks—Punjab Resource Management Programme and the Poverty Focused Investment Strategy (PFIS)—to tap into resources, technically assist with change, and help institutionalize reform. The PFIS served as the guiding framework with health as one of its areas.[91] Under its aegis, the Punjab Health Sector Reform Framework (HSRF) was developed in 2005.[92] The model of restructuring First Level Care Facilities (FLCFs) adopted under the HSRF was centred on directly-managed services with increased funding as opposed to the earlier models, which were built around contracting out; these have been described in detail in a subsequent section. In addition, the Punjab Devolved Social Services Programme,[93] also focused on health through work in the inter-sectoral domain. However, it must be noted that all these healthcare reform-related initiatives in Punjab stretched the already over-committed technical workforce. Lack of planned technical assistance is, therefore, recognized as one of the major impediments to health reform within the province.[94,95]

As opposed to NWFP and Punjab, there is no named reform unit either in Sindh or in Balochistan. In both the provinces, however, the PHC contracting out model was implemented, as has been described later in this chapter. In Sindh, initiatives for grant of autonomy to the three major hospitals and appointment of a special secretary to oversee major preventive programmes are additional systems reform related attempts.

1.3.3 History of reform initiatives at the Primary Health Care level

Primary Health Care in Pakistan comprises curative and preventive services—the latter as part of the national public health programmes delivered through FLCFs and community workers. The foundation of FLCFs in Pakistan was laid by the Bhore Committee Report in 1946, a year before the country was created.[96] After Alma Ata and during the 1980s, the state healthcare delivery system as a whole was reoriented towards the implementation of PHC.[97] By the end of the 1980s, Pakistan had more than 12,000 FLCFs. However, issues with their performance were widely recognized.[98] Since then, several efforts have aimed to reform their management. In the early 1980s, the World Bank's Family Health Project was launched to facilitate health facility upgradation.[99] Under the project, District Health Development Centres were created all over the country. These serve as a sustainable institutional mechanism to build capacity of many categories of healthcare providers at the district level, to this date. Although many publications refer to the Family Health Project, formal evaluations of this project are not available in the public domain. Later, management reforms were introduced—during the 1990s—under the Social Action Programme (SAP). These reforms failed to yield the desired impact due to a number of reasons.[100,101] The attempt to decentralize the healthcare system within a centralized government system was one of the reasons. The issue remains unresolved even after the formal decentralization of government in 2001.

More recent management restructuring arrangements have involved contracting out management of FLCFs to NGOs. Since then, reform of FLCFs has generated both political interest as well as controversy. The institutional history of reform in this area is rooted in the Lodhran initiative. This was a PHC management restructuring arrangement, which involved contracting out management of Basic Health Units (BHUs) to a parastatal NGO in one union council—a sub-district level—in 1999.[102] The model was expanded as the Chief Minister's initiative in 12 districts of the country as the Rahim Yar Khan project in 2003.[103] Shortly thereafter, it was up-scaled nationwide to 30 per cent of Pakistan's districts as the President's Primary Health Care Initiative.[104] Since the change in government in 2008, the programme has been labelled as the People's Primary Health Care Initiative.[105] The programme's weaknesses were not fully factored into planning while up-scaling the model to the national level under the President's high-level initiative. Additionally, as the programme remained outside of the departments of health and was managed by the Ministry of Special Initiatives, the health community remained reluctant to own the model. Turf rivalries, therefore, led to the concomitant introduction of another model in the Punjab province. This model was centred on improving directly-managed services within public sector management arrangements and the introduction of measures to benchmark performance through the development of Minimum Service Delivery Standards.[106,107] Both the reform initiatives have shown initial process level success.[108,109] However, lessons learnt from them have not been systematically analyzed to develop a consolidated policy for reform of PHC.

1.3.4 Public health, water and sanitation: A historical snapshot

After the creation of Pakistan in 1947, tropical disease control programmes characterized public health. In the late 1980s and 90s, a range of vertical disease-specific national programmes were introduced in Pakistan by international agencies. These programmes include the national programmes for immunization and nutrition and programmes aimed at prevention and control of malaria, tuberculosis, and HIV and AIDS. Later, a more organic crop of national programmes focusing on MCH and others aimed at prevention and control of hepatitis, blindness, and non-communicable diseases (NCDs) were established. Non-governmental Organizations such as Sight Savers and Heartfile played a major role in lending impetus to the blindness and NCD programmes, respectively.[110,111] The NCD prevention and control programme was not fully institutionalized. Recently, efforts have been initialized to revitalize action in this area. However, the opportunity to build further on the work already done appears to have been missed.[112] Details about some of these programmes are provided in the chapter on *Service Delivery*. Since most of the existing disease-specific programmes are implemented at the level of FLCFs, poor performance at that level deeply impacts the ability of these programmes to deliver on stipulated targets. In addition, their vertical planning, management, and institutional arrangements have created many issues at the district level, where programmes are actually implemented. These issues have not received priority in health systems planning and reform. However, as global attention now shifts from diseases to health systems, the government will have to take the systems dimensions of these diseases into serious consideration.[113]

As opposed to prevention, health promotion has never been a priority area in public health in Pakistan except for its inclusion alongside prevention and control in the National Action Plan for the Prevention and Control of Non-Communicable Diseases and Health Promotion in Pakistan.[114] The lack of due attention to NCDs and health promotion represents a major weakness in Pakistan's public health planning. Similarly, other important areas such as occupational and environmental health have also been outside of mainstream public health planning.

Water and sanitation is the mandate of the lowest functional unit of the government and has, in theory, always been a priority in the government's five-year plans.[115] It was one of the four components of the Social Action Programme in the 1990s and more recently, has featured prominently on provincial social sector programmes and the Prime Minister's Poverty Reduction Programme.[116] Despite due emphasis on planning theoretically, the provision of clean water and adequate sanitation is a problem and diarrhoeal diseases continue to be the third leading cause of death in children.[117] In urban areas, corroded and broken pipes, which often connect with sewage and drainage pipes, are part of the problem and lead to frequent infectious disease epidemics.[118] Shortage of piped water additionally leads to the use of water from unhygienic sources. In the rural areas, geographic reasons and lack of access to piped water accounts for availability issues whereas in major cosmopolitan cities, tanker mafias create artificial shortages. The projected water scarcity is likely to further exacerbate these issues.[119] There have been ample resources at the local level for water and sanitation with responsibility fully devolved to local governments. However, as infrastructure building at the local level is fraught with many governance challenges with opportunities for corruption and pilferage, resources are poorly-targeted to develop the needed local solutions. On the other hand, the government's recent programme on safe water, entailing a significant investment in the installation of filtration plants all over the country, has very limited outreach. It is important to develop local community-suited solutions to safe water and adequate sanitation. Promoting transparency at the local government level to ensure effective targeting of resources is critical in this regard.

1.3.5 History of hospital reform

As the largest expenditure category, public hospitals account for more than 60 per cent of health spending by provincial health departments.[120] However, many public hospitals in Pakistan, as in rest of the developing world, have poor performance with respect to management and quality endpoints.[121] Over the years, successive governments have used hospital autonomy as a strategy to overcome these issues. In Punjab, autonomy was granted to 9 teaching and 16 other hospitals through the Punjab Medical and Health Institutions Ordinance in 1998, whilst an overarching process of reform was establishing the District Health

Authorities and the District Health Government systems. The process of hospital autonomy was supported by a World Bank Learning and Innovation Loan.[122] Legislation enabled appointment of Chief Executive Officers (CEOs) and Board of Governors, establishment of Institutional Management Committees (IMCs) and granting of financial and administrative powers. A few institutions were able to benefit from these arrangements. These were institutions with smaller administrative units, better physical infrastructure, and those that could develop satisfactory options for institution-based private practice for doctors, as in the case of the Punjab Institute of Cardiology.[123] Although there has been no robust evaluation of impact, it is widely perceived that most hospitals were unable to successfully restructure under the new arrangements due to a number of factors.

The North-West Frontier Province initiated the hospital autonomy reform process with technical assistance from the Asian Development Bank,[124] and support from German bilateral assistance. Under the NWFP Medical and Health Institutions Reform Act 1999, a new set of rules was stipulated to appoint CEOs, establish IMCs and grant limited financial autonomy, as in Punjab. These changes enabled a few hospitals to generate income and better manage their own staff.[125] However, desirable level of autonomy was not granted, given partial controls over financial arrangements and limited human resource administrative prerogatives of the CEO. This was complicated by patronage and rivalry among staff. All these experiences show that barring a few notable exceptions, hospital autonomy initiatives in Pakistan have generally led to gains in the area of revenues for hospitals and incentives for staff but have not been used as a tool to promote quality and equity.

As opposed to legislation, executive authority was used to replicate the success of one hospital in Sindh.[126] This lent impetus to the establishment of District Health Boards in all districts for district level Civil Hospitals and Hospital Management Committees for *Taluka* level hospitals. The approach is presently being strengthened through multilateral support.[127]

Institution-based private practice is the other institutional change lever within a hospital setting in the context of reform. Efforts to date in Pakistan have been bitter failures and evidence from them is usually not factored into subsequent planning.[128,129] In this connection, NWFP's experience with enacting legislation in 2001 can be regarded as the most controversial case in Pakistan. More recently in 2005, the federal government undertook measures to institutionalize institution-based private practice in response to the Supreme Court's proceedings on a human rights case.[130] As an outcome, the Ministry of Health articulated recommendations to develop a policy framework in a brief to the Prime Minister.[131] The framework has not been implemented, to date. The chapter on *Service Delivery* discusses other aspects of hospital reform in Pakistan.

1.3.6 History of health financing

In general, there have been limited efforts on part of successive governments to overcome the key disparity in health financing—the predominance of out-of-pocket payments as a means of financing health, as evidenced by data presented in Table 5 in the chapter on *Health Financing*. A few attempts have been made in the past to enhance revenue and donor allocations for health. Aggregate increases were made during the SAP years—in the 1990s—and later during the period 2002–2007.[132] However, allocations were not enough to meet needs and because of inattention to issues of utilization, were unable to create the desired impact.

Since the early 1990s, there have been repeated calls for developing alternatives to revenues as a means of health financing.[133] However, the potential therein has not been capitalized. Donor agencies have explored the potential within social health insurance but have not been able to fully institutionalize arrangements.[134,135] In NWFP, bilateral agencies have promoted social health insurance with support from the religious community, capitalizing its non-profit solidarity characteristics and have primed policy-makers to the need for action. However, this has not fully cascaded into implementation. The Federal and Punjab governments have constituted task forces from time to time to explore options but with no tangible outcomes.

Many initiatives have explored the potential to upscale Pakistan's existing system of social health protection. However, none has led to concrete action. As a result, there are minimal linkages between Pakistan's existing Social Protection Strategy and the health sector. During the design phase of the strategy, the Asian Development Bank, which provided technical assistance to the government for the project, envisaged five areas for the strategy. Social health insurance was one of these alongside social assistance, micro- and area-based schemes, child protection, and labour markets.[136] The development study of the project also included a component on health insurance, which recommended the introduction of a social health insurance scheme on a 'start small and grow' basis, financed by contributions as well as supplementary funding sources.[137] However, the final strategy document released in 2005 did not include health in its core instruments.[138] Social protection is the critical link to financing health for Pakistan's population in the informally employed sector and can be an important tool if dovetailed with exemption systems in public hospitals, most of which levy a user fee. Through this, a demand side financing strategy can be structured—an approach known to facilitate equitable access to healthcare.[139,140]

Many other health financing related missed opportunities can also be enumerated. The Employees Social Security Institute (ESSI)—details of which are given in chapter 2—presently accounts for 0.99 per cent of the total spending on health. The health sector has neither worked nor lobbied for legislation to secure a higher number of employees under this scheme. Health has also been unable to reap the benefits of the enabling environment created for the insurance industry through the Insurance Ordinance, 2000. With appropriate regulatory approaches and policies, private health insurance could have helped in promoting financial risk protection, at least for a segment of the country's population.[141] Similarly, the public sector has also not taken advantage of recent growth in the microfinance sector and the existence of infrastructure at the grass roots level, which can make community health insurance for the poor, commercially viable by offsetting administrative costs, as has recently been shown by pilot projects established by microfinance institutes.[142] The chapter on *Health Financing* discusses other opportunities and gaps in this regard.

1.3.7 Human resource and the health system: A historical snapshot

Pakistan has given much attention to increasing the number of doctors and medical schools over the last 62 years; as a result, the number of doctors has increased from a few hundreds in 1947 to over 127,000, as is presently documented.[143] However, medical education follows the clinical model with little emphasis on prevention, health promotion, or community involvement. Other categories of healthcare providers have also not received adequate attention, because of which there is an acute shortage of nurses, paramedics, dentists, laboratory and surgical assistants, management and public health experts, and midwives. Qualitative issues, high attrition rates, mal-distribution, and deployment issues and gaps at the level of training and capacity building are also well-established. In recent years, the focus has been on privatization of medical education, which has created many regulatory problems. As opposed to this, strategic approaches to capacity building, continuing medical education, and retention regulation have not been prioritized. The chapter on *Human Resource* discusses these further under *Health workforce* and the *Human resource dimension of health administration.*

Many cadres of community health workers have been introduced over the years. Most of these have not been subsequently consolidated, despite the opportunity provided by the establishment of District Health Development Centres as part of the Family Health Project in the 1990s. Pakistan established programmes for Traditional Birth Attendants and Lady Health Visitors in 1950 and 1975, respectively. Both were not provided adequate support and hence to this date, there is shortage of Skilled Birth Attendants (SBAs) in the country, with only 39 per cent of deliveries being assisted by them.[144] In 1988, the nationwide community-based Lady Health Workers (LHWs) programme was launched in a vertical federally-led design. Lady Health Workers are meant to provide door-to-door basic services in rural areas at the grass roots level. This is one of the few programmes, which has received consistent support from successive governments. In 2006, another cadre of community workers, the Village Based Population Health Workers of the Ministry of Population Welfare was merged with the LHW workforce. There are currently an estimated 90,000 LHWs delivering services in the field. Recently, the government has decided to increase the number of LHWs to 200,000 over the next five years.[145] As opposed to this quantitative target, qualitative issues of deployment and capacity and issues with the programme's vertical configuration have not been the focus of attention. Human resource issues have been discussed in detail in the relevant chapter.

1.3.8 Medicines and related products: A historical snapshot

The pharmaceutical sector was regulated by the Drug Act 1940 and the Pharmacy Act 1967 until 1972, which is when the Generic Drug Act was promulgated. The latter introduced a major change in the pharmaceutical sector. However, the act had to be repealed in the wake of strong opposition by the commercial sector and the medical community and was replaced by the Drug Act 1976, which currently regulates the pharmaceutical sector. In 1993, the National Drug Policy was pronounced—long after promulgation of the 1976 statute. Although both the act and the policy are technically robust in relation to many attributes, they also suffer from numerous limitations.[146] The Drug Act 1976, in particular, has not been updated since the enunciation of the World Trade Organization's (WTO) statutes and Pakistan's Patent Ordinance 2000. As a result, rules and guidelines, which can enable Pakistan to make use of flexibilities permissible under WTO to protect public health, have not been framed.

The chapter on *Medicines and Related Products* alludes to many other weaknesses of the law in the area of quality and price regulation. However, by far, the most important weakness of the Drug Act 1976 and National Drug Policy 1997 relates to their implementation, which creates space for manoeuvrability and exploitation. The resulting abuse leads to compromised quality and higher prices of drugs. Problems at the level of implementation can be complicated further by the issuance of Statutory Regulatory Orders, which create confusion and unevenness in the application of policies. It is also important to appreciate that medical devices, technologies and traditional medicines—areas fraught with high level of collusion in quality and/or price regulation—are currently outside of the ambit of law.

Price regulation is an important area; however, the Ministry of Health has not explored the potential within various approaches of differential pricing, bulk procurements, etc., to reduce prices of drugs. The only regulatory measure, which involved partial deregulation of prices of drugs in 1993, led to unprecedented increases in prices of drugs and was, therefore, abandoned.[147]

In 2005, after the issue of spurious drugs came into the spotlight subsequent to a *suo moto* action by the Supreme Court of Pakistan,

Cabinet approval was given for establishment of an independent Drug Regulatory Authority (DRA). However, progress in that area has not been evident. The chapter on *Medicines and Related Products* discusses these and many other considerations, in detail.

1.3.9 Health information systems: A historical snapshot

Over the years, investments have been made in setting up many health information systems in the country. These include a vital statistics sample surveillance system,[148] the Health Management and Information System (HMIS),[149] several vertical disease surveillance systems such as the Lady Health Worker Management Information System and the Expanded Programme on Immunization Management Information System, and a range of periodic surveys.[150] Donors have played an active role in building capacity in line with their global role in supporting respective instruments. The United States Agency for International Development (USAID) has supported the Pakistan Demographic and Health Surveys (PDHS), the World Bank has promoted the Pakistan Social and Living Standards Measurement (PSLM) Survey and UNICEF has helped institutionalize the provincial Multiple Indicator Cluster Survey (MICS) system. The World Health Organization, on the other hand, has invested in building the polio surveillance system whereas the Canadian International Development Agency (CIDA) has supported high-risk surveillance of HIV and AIDS within the country. Recasting of HMIS and its transformation into the District Health Information System (DHIS), currently underway in many districts, is being supported through Japanese bilateral assistance. These information systems have the potential to yield meaningful evidence if some of their weaknesses are addressed. Specific details have been discussed in the relevant chapter.

In 2005, Heartfile lent impetus to and led an effort in collaboration with the Federal Bureau of Statistics and the Ministry of Health to review existing health information systems and develop recommendations aimed at bridging key weaknesses in this space.[151] Recommendations focused on bridging gaps within individual health information strands. Additionally, they called for the creation of an apex institutional structure, a data policy, a mechanism for periodically reporting on health indicators, and the optimal use of technology to streamline data flows.[152] The Federal Bureau of Statistics has followed up on these recommendations by creating a system of National Health Accounts and dedicating apex responsibility for annually collating health information on the pattern recently conducted. The Ministry of Health is yet to act on the recommendations in order to bridge gaps within individual data streams.

1.3.10 History of decentralization in Pakistan

Many attempts have been made in the past to decentralize the healthcare system, notably in the province of Punjab. Prior to 2001, Punjab initialized many decentralization reforms with multilateral support. In the early 1990s, financial management of health was decentralized to the *Tehsil* level; however, lack of capacity at the *Tehsil* level was largely responsible for the failure of this initiative.[153] The second decentralization attempt—the Sheikhupura Project—was pilot to the Second Family Health Project. The pilot aimed at creating a viable model for PHC and was introduced in a case control evaluation design as a management intervention study with decentralization of administration within districts, integration of existing vertically organized mono-purpose programmes, and community participation as its major components.[154] As the project was not fully owned by the administration, primarily as a result of opposition from departmental auditors, it was eventually abandoned. A formal evaluation of this project is not available in the public domain, and therefore lessons cannot be incorporated into health systems planning.

The third decentralization attempt was introduced in 1996/97. This involved the establishment of District Health Authorities (DHA) and District Health Management Teams (DHMT). The initiative followed the National Health Policy of 1997 and was part of the government's agenda to decentralize administration of public sector departments as envisaged by SAP II. Provincial and District Health Development Centres, which were established earlier under the Family Health Project, supported the initiative. District Health Authorities were established through executive order in the districts of Jhelum and Multan respectively, whereas DHMTs were established in 16 out of the 34 districts in Punjab. During this period, Punjab also promulgated the Punjab Medical and Health Institutions Ordinance 1998, under which autonomy was granted to its public hospitals, as has previously been described.

In 1998, the District Health Government (DHG) reform was introduced—the fourth attempt at decentralization. This entailed revamping the overall structure of the Department of Health of Punjab and separation of the Secretariat and Directorate within the department. The former was meant to be mandated in a normative and quality assurance role whereas the latter was supposed to be entrusted with implementation. The idea was to decentralize management to smaller management units. In addition, DHGs focused on purchaser-provider separation and intra-organizational contracting between the Department of Health as purchaser and the DHG as provider with the intention of introducing elements of competition as an incentive for improving performance and quality. The DHGs were also meant to include representatives from population and social welfare, and were therefore, oriented in an inter-sectoral scope. The DHG reform was eventually abandoned with the change of government in 1999. Some of its elements did, however, transition into the devolution initiative introduced two years later in 2001.

The local government initiative of 2001 involved devolution of political and administrative authority to Pakistan's 135 districts under the Local Government System.[155] The reform was envisaged to empower local communities and enhance government effectiveness but fell prey to turf rivalries between provinces and districts. Modification of statutes and procedures watered down the spirit of the law after its inception. The reform staggered half implemented during the period 2002–2009. In July 2009, three out of the four provincial governments indicated that they plan to revert administrative arrangements back to the pre-2001 system. The section on *Decentralization* in the chapter on *Institutional Reform* discusses this initiative in detail.

1.4 Lessons learnt

There are some important lessons to be learnt from the historical account of attempted healthcare restructuring presented in this chapter. First, it is important to appreciate that there have been many attempts in the past to bring about change in the health sector. Health systems restructuring has been promoted and supported more actively by multilateral financial institutions and some bilateral donors as opposed to WHO, which has played an important role in disease prevention and control. However, despite many attempts, there have been no efforts to promote a consolidated vision for reform and institutions such as the Ministry of Health, which could have spearheaded reform, have not invested in building capacity to mainstream transformational change.

Secondly, institutions also lack the capacity to monitor and evaluate and consolidate lessons learnt, and therefore, important earlier restructuring pilots such as the *Sheikhupura* pilot project and the DHA, DHMT, and DHG initiatives have remained poorly documented, with very little evidence in the public domain with respect to process level impediments, which could guide further efforts.

Thirdly, there appears to be no institutional memory or commitment to build on work in the pipeline and consolidate efforts underway. Successive governments have adopted options while subsequent governments have disregarded them. Information collated in this chapter, triangulated with the analysis summarized in subsequent chapters of Part II of this publication, indicates that it has almost become a given for those in political roles to prioritize planning based on what is politically expedient and those in administrative roles not to confront them because of the fear of undue accountability or complacency. The analysis indicates that the institutional environment is, therefore, increasingly getting focused on short-term gains as opposed to outcomes and politicization of decision-making, patronage, tolerance to circumventing procedures, systemic manipulation, and graft has become a norm. Those in technical and administrative roles in ministries and departments do not appear to have the voice, clout or tenure security needed to make it implicitly binding on incoming governments to conform planning and action with evidence. Consequently, every government starts *de novo* as plans in the pipeline are rolled back and technical assistance financed through loans fails to be targeted, resulting in significant wastage of the tax-payers' money and loss of confidence of international stakeholders. Regrettably, there is no mechanism in place to hold governments accountable for such actions.

Any effort to mainstream health reform must therefore proceed with a multi-stakeholder sign-up to an Agenda for Reform. An inclusive and participatory process should garner consensus of multipartisan stakeholders, development partners, the establishment, and the civil society on a technically viable roadmap for reform and structure multi-stakeholder oversight of the process of its implementation to ensure that reform outlives administrations and is not held hostage to short-term stakes. This is a critical prerequisite to any substantive action to implement reform.

Chapter 2

Health Systems in Pakistan

Contemporary health systems are difficult to categorize into various models, given their diversity, which stems from variations in the combination of financing and service delivery arrangements. That notwithstanding, if mechanisms to finance healthcare are taken as a yardstick, contemporary health systems fall into three broad categories. The first category includes welfare models. These are financed predominantly through public sources of health financing, which include revenues and/or pooling through payroll taxes or social security contributions. Examples include health systems of high-income countries of Western Europe, the Gulf Cooperation Council countries, and Canada. The second category, of which the United States of America is the prototype, is characterized predominantly by a market system of pooling and provision. Majority of the low- and middle-income countries including Pakistan fall within the rubric of the third category, where publicly financed government health delivery coexists with privately financed market delivery in a Mixed Health System.[156]

Before going on to describe the details of Pakistan's health system, the definitional context needs to be set forth. Traditionally, a health system is defined as 'comprising all the organizations, institutions and resources that are devoted to producing health actions.'[157] Part of the health system delivers personalized curative care or public health services, and therefore, gets labelled as a healthcare system. The World Health Organization describes the healthcare system as comprising six building blocks—service delivery, health workforce, information, medical products, vaccines and technologies; financing, and leadership and governance.[158] This publication additionally pitches technology as the seventh health systems domain on the premise that its potential to enhance efficiency and connectivity, and control errors and costs would bring value to a resource-constrained developing country.

It must be recognized, however, that a health system is much broader than a healthcare system. It is now well-established that factors influencing and determining health status at the individual and population levels can be socio-economic, environmental, biological, or lifestyle related in nature and that considerations relevant to population dynamics, human development, overarching governance, international and domestic politics, and security have a deep bearing on health status and healthcare delivery. These broader determinants, which can be modified through action in the inter-sectoral domain, have been discussed further in chapter 10 under *Social policy reform and health*. Recognizing the importance of these factors, this publication illustrates a health systems framework, which in addition to outlining the interaction between various health systems domains also demonstrates the impact of factors outside of the healthcare system in influencing health status (Figure 2). The annotations to Figure 2 indicate the means of assessing performance of the health system, as has been discussed later in this chapter.

2.1 Pakistan and its healthcare systems

Located in South Asia, Pakistan gained independence from colonial rule in 1947. As the sixth most populous country in the world, its current population stands at 160 million, 65 per cent of which lives in the rural areas,[159] 46 per cent of which is illiterate,[160,161] and 36.9 per cent below the age of 15 years.[162]

Pakistan has a parliamentary form of democracy; however, out of 62 years of its existence, the country has been under military rule for 31 years. Economic growth has been dependent on the level of international support, as opposed to democracy vs. military rule. Growth in the 1960s and 1980s can be attributed to strong US support; the latter in the wake of the Afghan war. In the 1990s, ending of the Afghan war and Pakistan's declaration of its nuclear capability led to plummeting of growth due to decline in development assistance. During the period 2001–07, debt rescheduling, and increase in foreign assistance and remittances subsequent to Pakistan's post-9/11 support to the 'war on terror' has been a strong factor leading to economic growth. However, growth could not be sustained. Despite these variations, there has been very little change in public sector allocations for health as a per cent of GDP over the last 62 years (Figure 3).[163,164]

Figure 2. The health systems framework

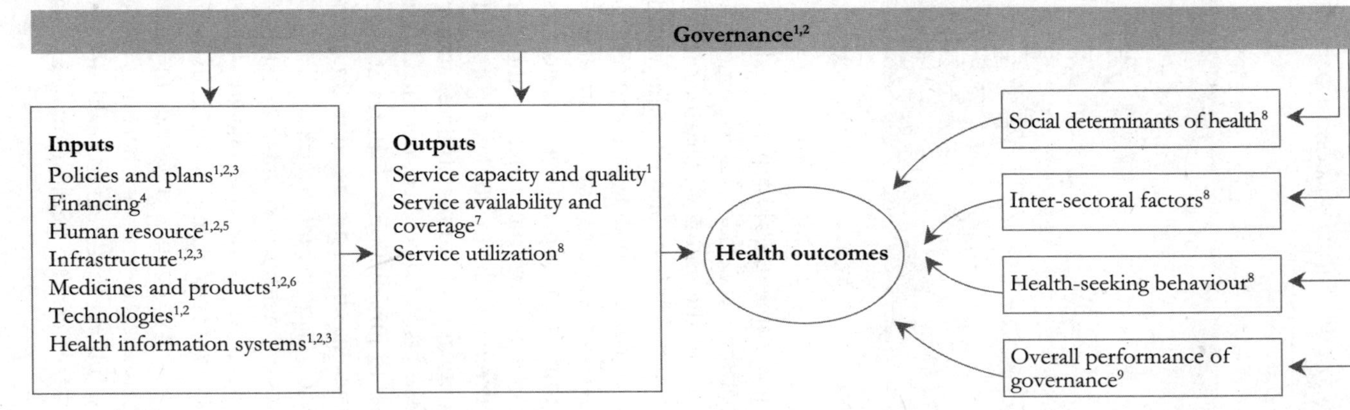

The footnotes indicate means of performance assessment

1. Periodic field surveys to assess performance against pre-defined indicators
2. Documentary and archival analysis
3. Annual reviews
4. National Health Accounts
5. Databases of administrative, regulatory, and accrediting agencies
6. Stock out rates
7. Management Information Systems
8. Pakistan Social and Living Standards Measurement surveys and Multiple Indicator Cluster Surveys
9. Cross-country performance assessments by international agencies

Figure 3. Government allocations for health as a percentage of GDP in the context of economic growth rate, during successive periods of military and democratic rule

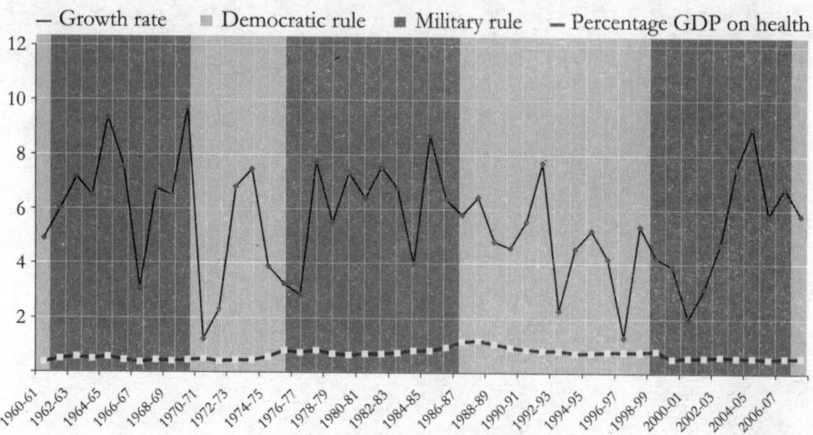

With respect to the form of government, Pakistan is a federating system with authority shared between the federal government and its four provinces;[165] 12.82 per cent of the country's territory is semi-autonomous and is under federal control.[166] Institutionally, the Ministry of Health is responsible for policy-making, coordination, and technical support. However, its role in providing services, both curative as well as preventive, has taken it away from its core normative functions as is discussed in the chapter on *Institutional Reform*, later in this publication. The provincial mandate is to deliver health. In 2001, as part of the government's reorganization, political and administrative authority was devolved to Pakistan's 135 districts.[167] Since then, decentralization of the government has fallen prey to jurisdictional disputes at several administrative and political levels, as has been discussed in the section on *Decentralization* in the chapter on *Institutional Reform*.

In relation to the healthcare system, within a country or territorial context, it is conventional to refer to a—or one—health system. However, if the functions of a health system are brought to bear—stewardship, financing, service delivery, human resource, medicines and related technologies, and information systems—it becomes evident that lumping together all the institutions that deliver health into one *system* may be misleading in Pakistan's context because many agencies delivering health in the country are vertically orientated. Here it is important to appreciate that this publication's denotation of *vertical* and *horizontal* is derived from the definition of these terms employed by the world of business science. Agencies that finance and provide/produce services for defined populations and have mutually exclusive governance and financing arrangements and means of harnessing inputs into the system have, therefore, been referred to as vertical in this publication. This definition has lent impetus to the understanding that a number of health systems exist in their own right in Pakistan. Of these, three can be described as truly vertical (Figure 4).

Figure 4. A stylized representation of healthcare delivery systems operating in Pakistan

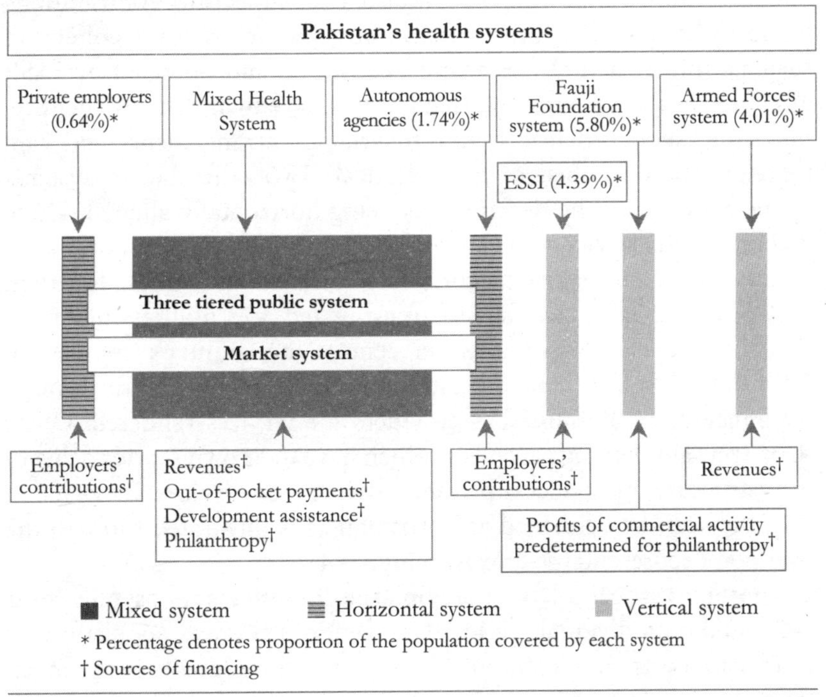

The Armed Forces health system is financed through tax revenues and has its own independent workforce, infrastructure, and governance arrangements. It provides health coverage to 6.29 million servicemen and their dependents. In the Fauji Foundation system, funds generated

by commercially viable non-profit conglomerates sustain a vertically integrated social protection system through which a range of social services including health are delivered to 9.1 million ex-military servicemen and their dependants. This accounts for 5.8 per cent of the country's population.[168] As in the previous case, the Fauji Foundation system has its mutually exclusive workforce and governance and service delivery arrangements. A similar situation is also seen for the Employees Social Security Institute (ESSI), a vertically-integrated health insurance system for the labour workforce in private industrial and commercial establishments with more than 10 employees under a stipulated salary scale. This is part of the Directorate of Labour and is, as such, totally outside of the purview of the departments of health.

More than 6.8 million individuals are secured under this scheme. The ESSI is financed through compulsory social security contributions made by employers. This autonomous system of fund collection sustains infrastructure and workforce owned and operated by ESSI. The three health systems described herein have their distinct clientele, financing, service delivery, and governance arrangements and can, therefore, be described as truly vertical. Two other health systems in the country can be described as being horizontally aligned. These include health services delivered by Pakistan's autonomous quasi-state organizations and Pakistan's corporate/commercial entities. Together, they provide health coverage to an estimated 3.73 million employees and their dependents or 2.38 per cent of the country's population. Both these systems finance health either by pooling for risk through insurance or by reimbursing providers for services rendered. Other than a few autonomous agencies, which have their own service delivery infrastructure, most access private providers for services. By virtue of this, they can be described as horizontal as is illustrated through the overlap of representative boxes in Figure 4.

The three vertical and two horizontal health systems almost fully cover 26.01 million individuals or 16.59 per cent of Pakistan's population for healthcare costs. However, outside of these arrangements is the much larger Mixed Health System characterized by roles played by public and private providers. This system provides healthcare coverage to 15.22 million employees of the government and members of the judiciary and legislature with general revenues as a means of financing. Additionally, 0.5 million individuals representing 0.32 per cent of the population are covered under safety net arrangements. With the inclusion of these in the afore-stated category of individuals in the country with health coverage, the total number of individuals covered for health stands at 41.73 million or 26.62 per cent of the country's population (Figure 5). The remaining 73.38 per cent of the population is not fully covered for health and predominantly seeks care by making out-of-pocket expenditures at the point of care in the Mixed Health System where the public and the market systems run in parallel. Notwithstanding frequent blurring of the line between the two—employees of the public system engage in dual practice as a conventional norm—the relative proportion of care delivered in the market system is predominant, as is evidenced by data from a cross-sectional nationally representative population-based survey (Figure 6).[169]

Figure 5. Pakistan's health systems—population receiving coverage for health (percentage)

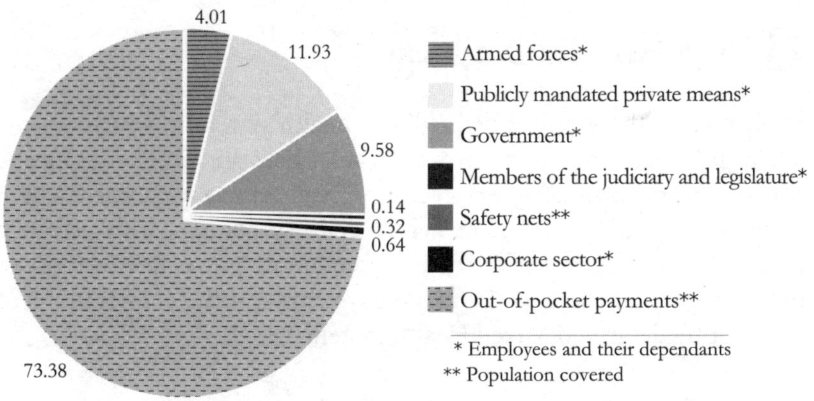

Figure 6. Access to healthcare services in the Mixed Health System

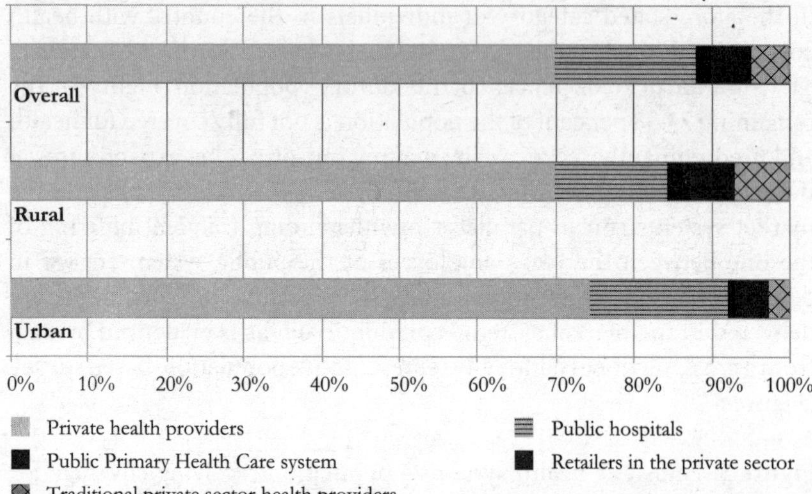

2.2 The Mixed Health System

A Mixed Health System is defined as 'a health system in which out-of-pocket payments and market provision of services predominate as means of financing and providing services, respectively in an environment where publicly financed government health delivery coexists with privately financed market delivery.'[170] The next section describes key features of both the public as well as the market systems and the connotations of the recently described Mixed Health System.

2.2.1 The public system

Pakistan's Mixed Health System has a strong post-colonial imprint with a 'national health services' model operating, albeit with several gaps. Revenues and development assistance finance the public system or the state's health infrastructure. This comprises the national public health programmes and three tiers of service delivery. The former, a set of disease-specific federally-led public health programmes are characterized by the federal government's leadership as the common denominator.

These programmes have varying levels of implementation autonomy within provinces and districts. Some of these are disease-specific such as the respective programmes on HIV and AIDS, malaria, tuberculosis, and hepatitis whereas others are cross-cutting. Key elements of each in terms of their scope and impact to date have been summarized in the chapter on *Service Delivery* (Figure 7).

Figure 7. Configuration of Pakistan's public healthcare system

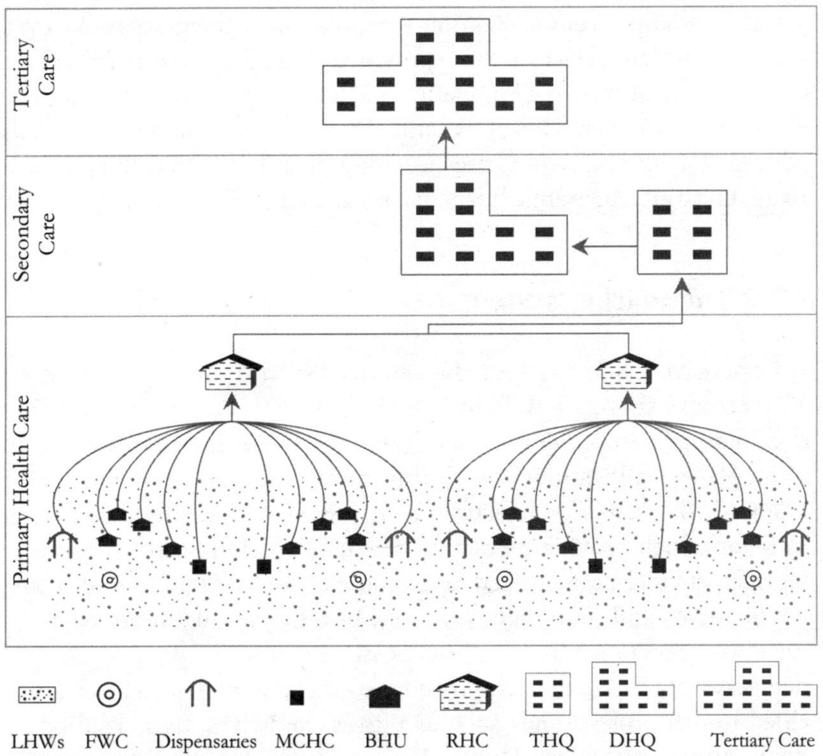

Basic Health Unit (BHU): a medical facility situated in the smallest administrative unit of government (Union Council) with an average catchment population of 10,000-20,000
Rural Health Centre (RHC): an upgraded PHC facility located at the sub-district administrative unit at the junction of four or five Union Councils; the population served ranges from 20,000-500,000
First Level Care Facilities (FLCFs): comprise BHUs and RHCs
Maternal and Child Health Centre (MCHC): MCH Centre of the Department of Health
Family Welfare Clinic (FWC): family planning facility of the Ministry of Population Welfare
Lady Health Worker (LHW): village-based female community health worker
Tehsil Headquarter Hospital (THQ): secondary level hospital
District Headquarter Hospital (DHQ): secondary level hospital

The physical infrastructure of PHC comprises many categories of service delivery outlets or FLCFs as shown in Figure 7. Over 12,000 FLCFs are meant to deliver basic clinical services in the country. Basic Health Units are also meant to deliver outreach services and serve as the implementation arm of the national public health programmes. However, more than 30 per cent FLCFs are currently non-functional despite efforts to restructure management of BHUs.[171] In addition, more than 90,000 community-based female Lady Health Workers provide preventive, maternal and child health, and related family planning services to 55 per cent of Pakistan's population at the grass roots level. Family planning services are also provided through 2740 Family Welfare Clinics of the Ministry of Population Welfare.[172] Secondary care includes *Tehsil* Headquarter Hospitals and District Headquarter Hospitals whereas tertiary care comprises teaching hospitals within the country. In all, there are 965 public hospitals in Pakistan.[173,174]

2.2.2 The market system

An extensive market system characterized by a diverse range of non-state actors exists alongside the public system in Pakistan and plays a dominant role in providing healthcare. The sector is heterogeneous in terms of the qualifications of healthcare providers, the system of medicine followed, the status of registration of providers, and the duration of time for which providers practice. The latter is significant since many service providers categorized as private are formally employed in the public sector and moonlight privately. In terms of qualifications, non-state providers range from doctors possessing modern western medical degrees or degrees in other approved medical systems to formally trained allied health professionals such as nurses, midwives, *dais*, Traditional Birth Attendants, Lady Health Visitors, Lady Health Workers, and untrained health providers. The latter is also a diverse group in its own right; most of them possess some form of training but are generally untrained for services they tend to offer. In the rural and peri-urban areas, paramedics pass off as doctors and laboratory technicians open laboratories, unsupervised. A range of faith healers also function within this environment; in the case of mental illnesses, faith healers are the most important cog in the pathways to care chain.[175] Furthermore, drug store operators, retailers, and unqualified sellers are also part of the landscape of informal providers.

With respect to the system of medicine followed, there is a clear dominance of modern western allopathic medicine. In addition, there are three different types of practices characterizing traditional medicine. These include *Tibb-e-Unani*, *Ayurvedia* and Homeopathy. According to recent data, 5 per cent of the total healthcare services are currently provided by practitioners of traditional medicine. Most of the qualified traditional health providers in various systems of medicine are registered with their own respective registration agencies.

A range of private sector healthcare facilities also characterize the market system. The *for-profit healthcare* sector includes ambulatory clinics operated by general practitioners or specialists, maternity homes, private dispensaries, diagnostic facilities, and private hospitals. There are a few large sophisticated private sector hospitals in major population centres. However, less than 10 private hospitals can be compared favourably with international hospital standards. Generally, the for-profit healthcare infrastructure is concentrated in major population centres. Since there has been no health facility census in the country to date and since there is no mechanism for registration of health facilities, it has not been possible to quantify the exact size of this sector and reach generalizable conclusions. Notwithstanding, nationally representative healthcare service utilization data previously shown in Figure 6, indicate significant predominance of private providers.

The *non-profit healthcare sector* comprises NGOs and charitable and trust-funded organizations. These are diverse entities providing a range of services. Pakistan's largest and most effectively functioning ambulance network is owned and operated by a charitable trust—the Edhi Foundation.[176] NGOs have traditionally played a significant role in delivering family planning services in Pakistan; the role of the Family Planning Association of Pakistan—now known as Rahnuma—is notable in this regard.[177] Non-governmental organizations have also been active more recently in the area of HIV and AIDS due to the availability of funds. Parastatal organizations such as the Rural Support Programmes have been involved in management restructuring of primary healthcare as is described in the chapter on *Service Delivery*. Other NGOs with a niche technical value have played important roles in their respective areas, such as in the case of Sight Savers, Heartfile and others. In addition, there are also a number of charitable hospitals in the country. According to a survey report compiled in 2005, there are an estimated 74 large charitable hospitals with over 7000 beds and hundreds of charitable clinics.[178] Additionally, many private sector hospitals also run significant charitable operations.

2.2.3 The Mixed Health Systems Syndrome

Despite the existence of a complex Mixed Health System, Pakistan has failed to achieve Health for All. This can be attributed to a number of factors, which have been described below. In relation to the healthcare system, the determinants of this failure are perceived to be rooted in the interplay of a *Triad of Determinants* recently described by the author—inadequate state funding, a burgeoning unregulated role of the private sector, and lack of transparency in governance in the Mixed Health System.[179] Figure 8 illustrates the dynamics of the relationship within the triad.

Chronic under-funding of the state's public health infrastructure is a major fault line. As a result, providers in the public system are seldom remunerated according to prevailing market trends. Better incentives in the private system lead to dual job-holding, and in remote areas, where oversight cannot be maintained, absenteeism and the ghost worker phenomenon become commonplace. Limited public resources also cannot sustain infrastructure of public facilities, as is evidenced by the state of dilapidation, most public facilities suffer from. To counter these limitations, administrations often impose user's fees, which in the absence of mechanisms to offset risk to the disadvantaged, can be detrimental to equity. In such an environment of under-provision and poor provision by the public sector, market mechanisms come into play to meet the ever-growing demand of burgeoning populations. The resulting out-of-pocket payments, coupled with rampant unethical provider behaviours—the latter because of gaps in regulation—undermine health systems performance. The situation is complicated further by rampant collusion in procurements, preferential treatment in staff deployment, and state capture by the elite, which biases norms towards issues to obtain selective benefits.

Figure 8. The public-private nexus in institutionalizing malpractices in the health sector

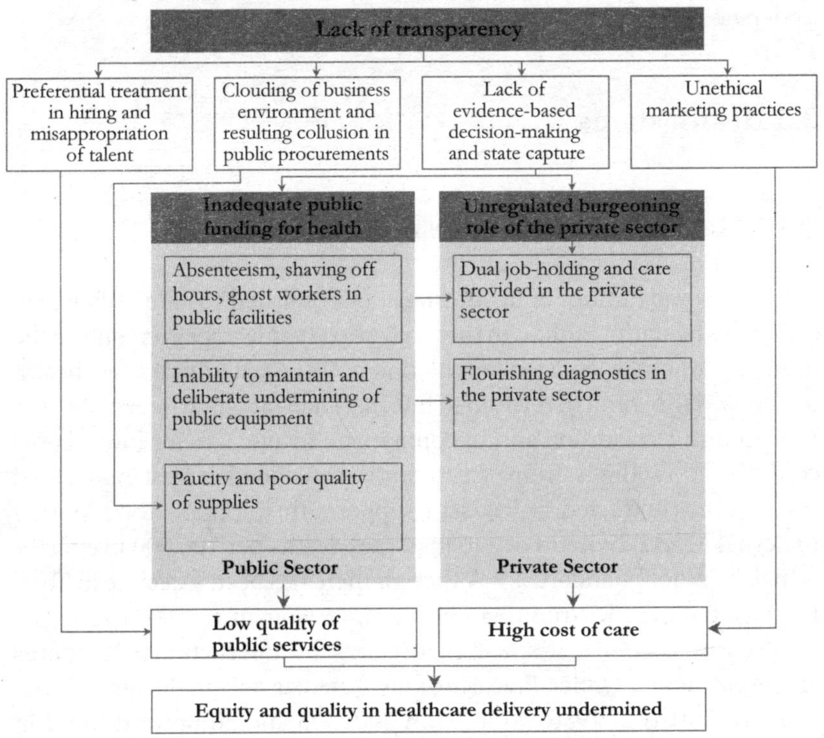

The public market interaction in the Mixed Health System and its manifestations, evidenced by compromised quality and equity in healthcare delivery, have been described as the Mixed Health Systems Syndrome—the denotation of syndrome refers to a set of concurrently appearing characteristics, which indicate poor performance with respect to key indicators of health systems performance. Limitations in achieving *fairness in financing* can be illustrated through the predominance of out-of-pocket payments as a means of financing health. The predominance of care provided by the private sector is evidence of management and performance issues in the public system and hence reflective poorly of *responsiveness*. In addition, inability to achieve *equity in outcomes* is endemic to these systems.

The public-private mix is not, however, a guarantee of poor performance. Locally relevant public policy choices can be adopted to develop stewardship mechanisms, which influence the behaviour of private providers in order to harness their outreach.[180] Many aspects of the reform agenda articulated in this publication hinge on this understanding.

2.3 Health status

2.3.1 Health status: A snapshot

The only compendium of health statistics published to date in Pakistan concludes by stating 'although there have been some improvements in the health status of the Pakistani population over the last 62 years, key health indicators lag behind in relation to international targets articulated in the Millennium Declaration and in comparison to averages for low income countries.'[181] Findings from the recently-concluded largest household survey ever conducted in Pakistan supports this notion—the reported Maternal Mortality Ratio of 276 maternal deaths per 100,000 live births is high by global standards.[182] Although there has been a decline in Total Fertility Rate (TFR) from 5.4 children per woman in 1990–91 to 4.1 children in 2006–07, it still remains high by international standards and even though Under-Five Mortality Rate has declined from 117 per 1000 live births in 1986–90 to 94 in 2002–06 and an upward trend in child immunization has been reported—increasing from 35 per cent in 1990 to 47 per cent in 2006—rates of improvements in health outcomes have been slow, particularly in comparison with other countries in the region.[183]

Pakistan also suffers from a number of other unique health challenges, particularly in relation to polio eradication and the prevention and control of NCDs, viral hepatitis and HIV and AIDS. Pakistan is one of the four countries of the world where polio has not been eradicated.[184] Recently, the prevalence of viral hepatitis in the general population has been reported at 7.4 per cent.[185] The double burden of disease and high prevalence of NCDs—more than 25 per cent of the population of the country suffers from one or more risk factors of non-communicable diseases—is also well established. Moreover, the recently reported 23 per cent prevalence of HIV and AIDS in high risk groups shifts the epidemic

Table 1. Pakistan's key health indicators

Health indicators	2005-06
Life expectancy (years)*	63.8[a]
Dependency ratio (per cent)*	68.7[a]
Crude Birth Rate (per 1,000)*	26.1[b]
Crude Death Rate (per 1,000)*	8.2[b]
Total Fertility Rate (children per woman)	4.1[c]
Contraceptive Prevalence Rate (per cent)	29.6[c]
Pregnant women receiving at least one ante-natal consultation (per cent)	61.0[c]
Women who receive care from Skilled Birth Attendants (per cent)	39.0[c]
Neonatal Mortality Rate (per 1,000)	54[c]
Infant Mortality Rate (per 1,000)	78[c]
Under-Five Mortality Rate (per 1,000)	94[c]
Fully-immunized children (per cent)	47[c]
Tuberculosis Case Detection Rate (per cent)	62[d]
Tuberculosis Case Detection Rate for new Sputum Smear Positive Cases (per cent)	49[d]
Tuberculosis Treatment Success Rate (per cent)	84[d]
Confirmed number of polio cases (as of 2 October 2009)	58[e]
Prevalence of viral hepatitis in the general population (per cent)	7.4[f]
Prevalence of smoking (over 18 years of age, per cent)	15.75[g]
Prevalence of leisure time physical inactivity (over 18 years of age, per cent)	91.5[g]
Prevalence of overweight and obesity (over 18 years of age, per cent)	38.5[g]
Prevalence of central obesity (over 18 years of age, per cent)	48.35[g]
Prevalence of high blood pressure (over 18 years of age, per cent)	13.7[h]
Prevalence of diabetes (over 25 years of age, per cent)	7.65[i]
Doctor-population ratio	1:1,326[g]
Nurse-population ratio	1:22,662[g]
Dentist-population ratio	1:3,039[g]
Households with toilet systems (per cent)	74[j]
Households with government garbage disposal services (per cent)	37[j]

* Estimations

a. Federal Bureau of Statistics, Pakistan. Pakistan Demographic Survey, 1998-2003
b. Federal Bureau of Statistics, Pakistan. Pakistan Population Census, 1998
c. National Institute of Population Studies and Macro International Inc. Pakistan Demographic and Health Survey, 2006-07
d. National TB Control Programme, Ministry of Health, Pakistan
e. National Expanded Programme on Immunization, Ministry of Health, Pakistan
f. Pakistan Medical Research Council, Ministry of Health, Pakistan; unpublished data
g. Heartfile, Ministry of Health and Federal Bureau of Statistics. Gateway Paper II: Health Indicators of Pakistan, 2007
h. Pakistan Medical Research Council, National Health Survey of Pakistan, 1994
i. Diabetic Association of Karachi and WHO surveys, 1994-1998
j. Social Audit of Governance and Delivery of Public Services Pakistan, 2005

scenario of the country to the concentrated epidemic level.[186,187] These data illustrate the emergence of additional challenges in the health sector. Pakistan's key health indicators have been summarized in Table 1.

2.3.2 Factors leading to poor health status

Health is an inter-sectoral responsibility. A number of factors are, therefore, responsible for poor health status of the country's population. These include the following:

Broader issues implicit in the social determinants: inequities in daily living conditions are an important determinant of health status.[188] With more than 25 per cent of the population of Pakistan living below the poverty line of less than US $1 a day and 46 per cent illiterate, the country suffers an inherent disadvantage in this regard.[189] Undernutrition is also highly prevalent with 36.8 per cent, 13 per cent and 38 per cent children stunted, wasted, and underweight, respectively.[190] This is likely to exacerbate as a result of the ongoing food security issues, inflationary pressures in view of Pakistan's recent economic downturn, and the global financial and commodity crises.[191]

Poor governance: malpractices and corruption are recognized within health systems globally,[192,193] and are known to have an independent negative effect on health outcomes.[194] On the other hand, evidence shows that a decline in corruption can improve health outcomes by increasing the effectiveness of public expenditure.[195] In contrast to this, data from many comparative country rankings show that public sector management and institutional governance are weak in Pakistan,[196,197] and that malpractices are widely prevalent in the health system.[198,199] Issues of governance and corruption have been identified as one of the key impediments to leveraging the potential within Pakistan's extensive health infrastructure.[200,201]

Low public investments in the health sector: public sector spending on health amounts to US $8.86 per capita, per annum in Pakistan, according to estimates presented in this publication. Low spending cannot sustain public infrastructure and leads providers to offer services in the private sector, thus acting as one of the three determinants of mayhem within Pakistan's health system, as has been described earlier in this chapter. Capacity to utilize funds is additionally low with poor quality of utilization.[202,203]

Factors in the inter-sectoral domain: many factors such as clean water, solid waste disposal, food security, occupational health and safety, safer working and general environments, and safe neighbourhoods are important for health status achievement but are not within the remit of the health sector. The large burden of diarrhoeal diseases in children in Pakistan is known to be closely related to the lack of sanitation facilities and safe sources of potable water.[204] Over the age of 65 years, 14 per cent of the rural females suffer from obstructive pulmonary disease,[205] which shows that the use of coal and biomass fuel to cook indoors is an important determinant of disease. Additionally, climate change is likely to further worsen the health impact of droughts and floods. Both these factors, particularly the latter, already cause significant mortality in Pakistan.

Political factors, conflict, and disaster: the overall political and security situation in a country has a deep bearing on health status. The recent conflict and extremism in Pakistan has claimed more lives than deaths from maternal and child health and HIV and AIDS combined in one year,[206] whereas an earthquake in 2005 claimed more than 75,000 lives. The determinants of failure to achieve polio eradication demonstrate the crucial role played by factors such as lack of access in a conflict-ridden zone, in undermining the effectiveness of public health interventions. As a result, Pakistan is one of the four countries in the world, where polio has not been eradicated to date.[207]

Poor performance of the health system: the performance of a health system can be gauged by the extent to which it enables achievement of three endpoints or goals. These include improving health status, financial risk protection, and ensuring responsiveness. Although an assessment of health systems performance has not been formally conducted, there is evidence from existing data of poor performance in relation to all the three endpoints. This has already been alluded to, whilst illustrating the characteristics of the Mixed Health Systems Syndrome.

The health status snapshot articulated earlier in this chapter is evidence of poor health status of the country's population. Lack of equity in health outcomes is additionally evidenced by inter- and intra-district disparities in outcomes.[208,209] Lack of fairness in financing can be illustrated through data presented in the chapter on *Health Financing*—73.38 per cent of the population of the country is not fully covered for healthcare costs. Even in the absence of formal measures to gauge responsiveness, management and performance issues discussed in the chapter on *Service Delivery* provide evidence of gaps in this area.

A formal health systems performance assessment is currently underway in Pakistan. The analysis is being conducted by Heartfile, using the mixed methods approach. Methods include analysis of existing data, archival and documentary reviews, and a field survey using structured and semi-structured questionnaires. The means of performance assessment have previously been illustrated in Figure 2. In addition to the establishment of a mechanism for periodic performance assessment of Pakistan's health system, the approach is envisaged to provide inputs to develop a standardized approach to measures, methods, and instruments as part of a WHO-led Platform to Strengthen Monitoring and Analysis of Country Health Systems. As such, Pakistan will serve as tracer country. Process insights and evidence from the approach adopted will help to develop a generic framework in order to assist with health systems performance assessment in the developing countries.

Part II

Health Systems Domains—a Review

The complexity of health systems has been described as being analogous to a 'black box' or a 'black hole.'[210] Analysis of individual health systems domains in Part II of this book will attempt to bring clarity to issues and outline a vision for reform in each domain.

CHAPTER 3

Health Governance

The viability and success of reform within any state sector is closely dependent on overall governance effectiveness and institutional ability to mainstream change. Reform of governance must, therefore, be a priority before reform in any other health systems domain is envisaged, particularly in view of the dismal state of overall and health governance in the country.

Reform of governance is one of the most difficult state reforms because of the inextricable relationship of governance with politics. Governance reform is only partly technocratic; it is largely a political process, both in terms of setting policy directions as well as reforming the public management process. Politicians and power-holders engage in governance reform in response to their own political interest and see it as a way of winning support, building or breaking coalitions, and reshaping the dynamics of political influence. An envisaged governance reform must be based on a sophisticated understanding of these political dynamics. This chapter will attempt to bring clarity to these considerations.

3.1 Concept, context, and actors

First of all, it is important to review the context in which the term governance is being used herein. Governance operates in organizations of any size—the government at several levels, businesses, corporations, NGOs, partnerships—or any other purposeful activity. It can also have several connotations—corporate governance, global governance, national governance, local governance, etc. However, the context in which governance is being used herein refers to *governance within government agencies* at various levels of the government system—federal, provincial, and local.

In this particular sense, governance is the subject of many interpretations and an amalgamation of many concepts; several expressions have been coined to describe the term. The World Bank scopes governance within the 'policy making and implementation' realms and includes 'accountable use of public resources and regulatory power' within the ambit of its definition.[211,212] The World Health Organization focuses on the concept of 'stewardship' and emphasizes the importance of 'oversight and guidance, on behalf of the state and its citizens.'[213] The United States Agency for International Development (USAID) regards it as a 'public management process.' The United Kingdom's Department for International Development, in its definition, underscores the importance of 'how systems of the state operate and relate to individual citizens,'[214] whereas UNDP lays emphasis on 'exercise of authority.'[215] By placing an emphasis on results management philosophies, the Paris Declaration on Aid Effectiveness and the more recently launched Accra Agenda emphasize the use of governance as a public management tool.[216,217] In addition, other definitions and norms of governance assessment have also been coined.[218]

This publication envisages governance as embodying a very broad concept—one that involves both policy making as well as implementation, or in other words, the development of rules and how rules apply; the concept also encompasses normative and instrumental aspects and deals with the exercise of authority at the economic, administrative, and political levels. In addition, the concept of governance as is being referred to herein, has both a strong institutional as well as an interface connotation. With reference to the latter, it takes into account the interaction between governance actors, whether they are individuals, groups or institutions and the relation of public service to the people. The discussion on health governance in this publication particularly focuses on the public management process and the cycle of public service efficiency and related issues of capacity, performance, and accountability.

Within the afore-stated paradigm, domestic health governance principally involves three sets of actors within Pakistan's Mixed Health System—state actors, health providers, and beneficiaries.[219] State actors include stakeholders in the public sector within and outside of the health system. In Pakistan's context, the former category includes the ministers and secretaries of health, the civil and technical bureaucracy, other staff at the federal, provincial and district levels, and human resource in administrative roles in health and related facilities. At an institutional level, the Ministry of Health, the provincial departments of health, and the offices of the Executive District Officers (EDOs), regulatory bodies and autonomous agencies and other state institutions described in the chapter on *Institutional Reform* fall within this category. At the political level, state actors include committees of parliamentary oversight. Public actors beyond the health sector, which have a role in shaping the sector, include the Ministry of Finance, the Planning Commission, public employee unions, public procurement and distribution agencies, and insurance companies. Vertical health systems described in the chapter on *Pakistan's Health Systems* have their own corresponding governance actors. The second set of actors includes health service providers in the state and non-state sectors. Details have been outlined in the chapter entitled *Health Systems* in Pakistan. The third set of actors includes the beneficiaries; these can be classified on the basis of income, location or by the category of services needed.

Many factors other than conventional actors also influence health governance. The role of media, political parties, advocacy and human rights organizations, civil society watchdogs, think tanks, and businesses in influencing governance is well recognized. In Pakistan's situation, particularly in the local government realm, landlords, land mafias, religious groups and other factions also shape the societal political culture and hence influence governance. All these governance actors interact in a highly complex manner within various streams of health systems.

Just as it is difficult to define governance, it is also difficult to categorize its domains. This publication classifies health governance into three domains: *Setting strategic directions, Implementation and oversight* and *Regulation*, with transparency and participation as cross-cutting themes. Table 2 categorizes currently used indicators, principles, and norms in health governance under these three areas to show that the classification being coined is all-embracing. Figure 9 builds on this further to outline additional domains whereas Table 3 elaborates on the roles of the public and private sectors in institutionalizing malpractices within these domains. It is evident from the description in the following chapters that most of the health systems maladies stem from problems in one of these three domains.

Table 2. Categorization of published health governance attributes under the domains of governance coined by this publication

Areas of governance (source: author)	Categorization of UNDP's principles, World Bank's indicators, WHO's domains and PAHO's essential health functions
Setting strategic directions	Generation of intelligence[1] Formulating strategic policy direction[1] Ensuring tools for implementation[1] Ensuring a fit between policy objectives and organizational structure and culture[1] Development of policies and institutional capacity for planning and management in public health[2] Direction (strategic vision)[3] Legitimacy and voice (participation and consensus)[3]
Implementation and oversight	Public health surveillance[2] Evaluation and promotion of equitable access to necessary health services[2] Monitoring, evaluation, and analysis of the health situation of the population[2] Performance (responsiveness, efficiency, and effectiveness)[3] Government effectiveness[4]
Regulation	Strengthening the institutional capacity for regulation and enforcement in public health[2] Regulatory burden[4]
Accountability	Ensuring accountability[1] Accountability and transparency[3] Voice and accountability[4] Control of corruption[4]
Participation	Building coalitions/building partnership[1] Social participation in health[2] Participation and consensus orientation[3]

1 World Health Organization
2 Pan American Health Organization
3 United Nations Development Programme
4 The World Bank

Table 3. Role of the public and private sectors in institutionalizing malpractices in the health sector

Areas and activities vulnerable to malpractices	Possible malpractices in the public sector *(and responsible stakeholder)*	Corresponding malpractices in the private sector *(and responsible stakeholder)*
1. Strategic vision and planning		
Development of plans, policies, and laws and allocation of resources	State capture *(politicians and decision-makers)*	Undue influence *(well-connected individuals and lobby groups)*
Administrative and regulatory norms and pronouncements	Impromptu orders (e.g. SROs), with resulting opaqueness and variance in the application of policies *(politicians and decision-makers)*	Undue influence *(well-connected individuals and lobby groups)*
2. Administrative decision-making		
Human resource hiring and placements	Preferential treatment to well-connected individuals and facilitative placements *(decision-makers)*	Undue influence *(well-connected individuals and lobby groups)*
Public procurements	Collusion in bidding and contracting *(decision-makers)* Record falsification, padding bills, over-invoicing and clever book-keeping *(administrative staff)*	Unethical incentives *(contractors and suppliers)* Planned substandard manufacture of consignments for the public sector *(manufacturers)*
Administrative approvals in public facilities	Receiving unauthorized payments *(administrative staff)*	Petty bribes for administrative clearance *(vendors and suppliers)*
3. Oversight of publicly financed and provided services		
Service delivery	Absenteeism and shaving-off hours, siphoning patients to private clinics *(providers of healthcare in the public sector)*	Disproportionate allocation of time to practice in the private sector *(staff qualified to practice)* Unauthorized practices; e.g., impersonating doctors *(staff not qualified to practice)*
Service prices (user fee)	Recieving unauthorized payments *(service delivery staff)*	Under the table payments *(patients)*
Supplies and stocks	Theft of supplies, pilferage, and dispensing to ghost patients *(store and procurement officers)*	Buy back in the market *(retailers and wholesalers)*

Continued...

Table 3. Continued...

Areas and activities vulnerable to malpractices	Possible malpractices in the public sector *(and responsible stakeholder)*	Corresponding malpractices in the private sector *(and responsible stakeholder)*
4. Regulation		
4.a Services in the private sector		
Permission to establish healthcare facilities	Non-existence of a comprehensive regulatory framework for the private sector	Mushrooming of health facilities without regard for quality or standards *(health providers and owners)*
Permission to establish pharmacies	Preferential treatment *(decision-makers)*	Undue influence to shape decision-making *(aspiring owners)*
Licensing, quality standards, and accreditation	Non-existence of a comprehensive regulatory framework for the private sector	Inattention to quality of care and malpractices *(healthcare providers and owners of private facilities)*
Output-based control of service prices	Non-existence of a comprehensive regulatory framework for the private sector	Stipulating fees without regard to access issues *(health providers and owners of private facilities)*
4.b Medical education		
Permission to establish facilities and numbers entering medical schools	Preferential treatment *(decision-makers and self-regulators)*	Undue influence to shape decision-making *(aspiring owners)*
Licensing, quality standards, and accreditation	Deliberate inattention to oversight in the case of non-compliance *(regulatory agencies)*	Undue influence to shape decision-making *(owners)*
4.c Human resource		
Licensing and credentialing	Self-serving regulatory capture *(regulators)*	Promotion of regulatory capture *(peer regulators with vested interest)*
4.d Pharmaceuticals		
Registration	Unnecessary registrations and IPR violations *(regulators)*	Unethical incentives *(manufacturers, traders, and wholesalers)*
Price regulation	Collusion in import tariffs and over-estimation in price calculations *(regulators)*	Unethical incentives and over-invoicing of raw material price *(manufacturers)*

Continued...

Table 3. Continued...

Areas and activities vulnerable to malpractices	Possible malpractices in the public sector *(and responsible stakeholder)*	Corresponding malpractices in the private sector *(and responsible stakeholder)*
Production and quality regulation	Deliberate inattention to oversight in the process of inspections *(inspectors and regulators)*	Import of low-quality raw materials *(importers and manufacturers)* Production of low-quality drugs or compliance with the lowest quality standards *(manufacturers)*
Regulation of wholesaling	Selling back pre-marked consignments to wholesalers in the market *(administrative staff)*	Buying back and resale of consignments; hoardings; unethical incentives to unduly influence decision-making; black market interplay *(wholesalers)*
Regulation of retailing	Deliberate inattention to oversight for non-compliance with standards *(regulators and inspectors)*	Fake licenses; absence of warranty of purchase; black market interplay; inadequate storage practices; unqualified staff; promotion of low-quality items; unethical incentives *(retailers)*
Regulation of marketing	Poor implementation of current norms of marketing; gaps in standards *(regulators)*	Unethical marketing practices *(non-bonafide pharmaceutical companies, wholesalers, importers, and traders)*

Figure 9. Domains of health governance

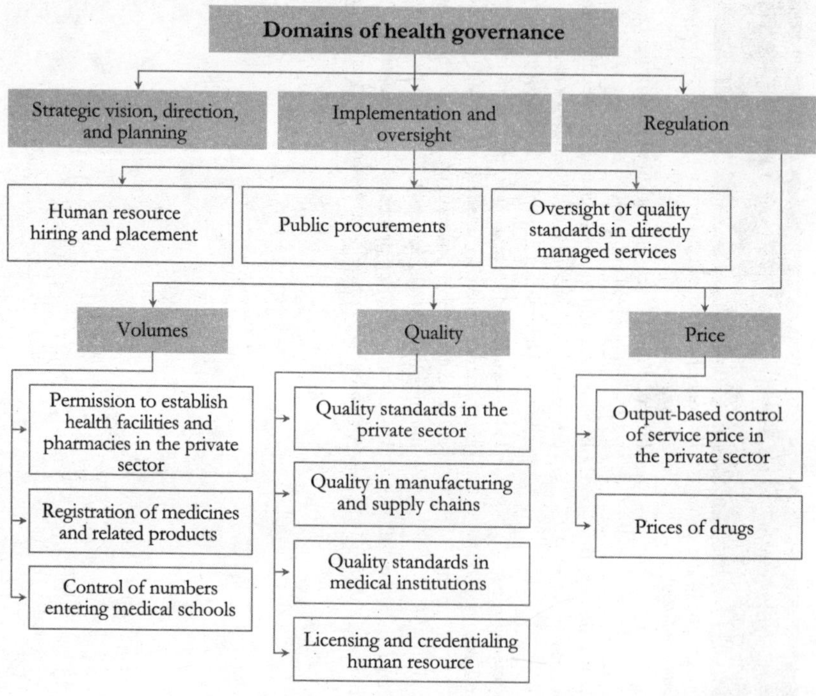

3.2 Domains of health governance

3.2.1 Setting strategic policy directions

There are many overlapping concepts in governance. Stewardship vis-à-vis governance is one of them. *Stewardship* in the context of the health sector refers to oversight and guidance on behalf of the state and its citizens, of the working and development of the nation's health actions whereas *governance* covers how authority over health resources and services is exercised.[220] Authority can have many dimensions in its own right, e.g., line managerial authority, monitoring authority, technical authority, coordination authority, supervisory authority, etc.[221] Stewardship can be considered synonymous with setting strategic directions; the latter includes developing a long-term vision, policy-making and establishing norms and standards. There are three issues relevant to this discussion—capacity limitations, weaknesses in accountability mechanisms, and gaps in transparency. As an outcome of these gaps, policies and plans often lack an outcome orientation and have limited grounding in evidence.

Capacity limitations exist at several levels in relation to stewardship functions. At the political level, health officials generally lack appropriate technical capacity to argue effectively for resources, get health issues on the political agenda, and set the needed strategic directions. At the civil service level, there exists what can be described as the colonial-contemporary lag. Pakistan's civil and administrative services have a strong post-colonial imprint and are, as such, geared to administrative control and exercising authority. A paradigm shift is needed so that participatory governance can enable harnessing all possible resources of the country to meet development goals.

Institutionally, at the technical level, there is limited capacity within agencies mandated in a stewardship and oversight role in health. These include the Ministry of Health and the provincial health and planning departments. However, it would be both difficult as well as inappropriate to generalize this statement because of inter- and intra-provincial variations in capacity to strategically plan and implement. Significant investments have been made through various initiatives, in particular WHO's Tropical Disease Research (TDR) programme and the Family Health Project to fund scholarships for postgraduate studies in various health systems streams over the past several decades. However, state agencies have not been able to retain most of the trained human resource due to inadequate incentives, poor working conditions, and lack of appropriate retention policies.

Capacity limitations manifest themselves in inability to plan strategically based on locally suited priorities and ultimately create space for decisions to be inadvertently donor driven. Additionally, policies remain focused on *processes* and *outputs* as opposed to *outcomes*, as has been the case with successive health policies of 1990, 1997 and 2001. As a result of limited capacity, the Ministry of Health and the departments of health do not perform their core essential functions and remain focused on peripheral and largely administrative issues. Essential functions, which merit attention as a priority—generation, collation, and interpretation of health-related information for policy and planning, setting norms and standards, regulation, quality assurance, and multi-sectoral action for health—therefore remain fragmented and unfulfilled. Institutional capacity gaps have been discussed further in the chapter on *Institutional Reform*.

Accountability is the unifying thread in governance. As a relationship, accountability should be a bridge between the stewards of health and citizens, and between health providers and the stewards of health. Within this context, accountability can be defined within political, performance, and financial realms.

At the political level, there are major gaps in direct and indirect political accountability. As a result of weaknesses in the former, politicians rarely press health-mandated agencies to pursue objectives and employ resources so that health providers become responsive to citizens' needs. Instead, priorities are determined by political expediency, whereas as a result of limited indirect political accountability, public sector health officials are usually not fully accountable to political actors.

Due to limited rational accountability of the decision-making process, policies and plans often have limited grounding in evidence. Evidence generally points to the need for long-term remedial measures. However, a combination of factors—lack of institutional memory, career structures that foster orientation around short-term outputs, and the tendency to focus on visible interventions—prevent evidence-based enduring actions from taking root. Additionally, there is no mechanism in place to make it binding on incoming governments to base decisions on evidence, and consolidate and strengthen existing initiatives. The chapter on *Structural Reform of the State and Health* focuses on transparency and accountability promoting measures to address these issues.

Lack of transparency in setting strategic directions can manifest itself in a range of ethical, intellectual, procedural, and financial forms of malpractices. Here, it is important to make a distinction between administrative malpractices/corruption and state capture. While administrative corruption takes many forms as has been described later, state capture is a manifestation of a broader systems phenomenon in policy and decision-making, where the laws of the land and policies are made to favour a few and those with vested interest and influence shape state policies, laws, and regulations. The challenge lies not only in the formulation of policies and laws but also in their application. Statutory Regulatory Orders and gazette notifications, which confer enormous powers of discretion, are a particular problem in this regard as they can create opaqueness in interpretation and variance in application of policies.

As a broad systems phenomenon, state capture is detrimental to the equity objective. However, in many cases, its existence is hard to prove. It has frequently been cited that the tendency to invest in civil works, physical infrastructure, and equipment purchases in health is motivated by vested interest. However, this may not always be the case. There could be several other reasons for the preference to invest in these areas. For example, decision-makers in the health sector with limited technical capacity may think that this is the best use of resources in health, and politicians, in their quest for interventions with quick visible results, may be inclined to invest in these areas to enhance their visibility. These factors need to be taken into consideration while deriving conclusions about the motivation behind decisions concerning resource allocations.

3.2.2 Implementation and oversight

3.2.2.i Public management process

Effective implementation, oversight, and regulation are critically dependant on the robustness of the public management process. The cycle in Figure 10 outlines attributes of the process. Core competency and capacity are a necessary prerequisite for public management. This can be ensured to a large extent though merit-based recruitments. Appropriate placements, clearly defined career paths, and performance-based incentives can be positive, motivationally. An enabling environment can be conducive to performance whereas appropriate oversight and accountability can counter collusion. Weaknesses in these attributes can lead to poor performance and inefficiencies and pave the way for collusion in public management in addition to fostering attitudinal maladies, which can lead public servants to please their superiors rather than be responsive to citizens' needs.

Figure 10. The Public Management Cycle

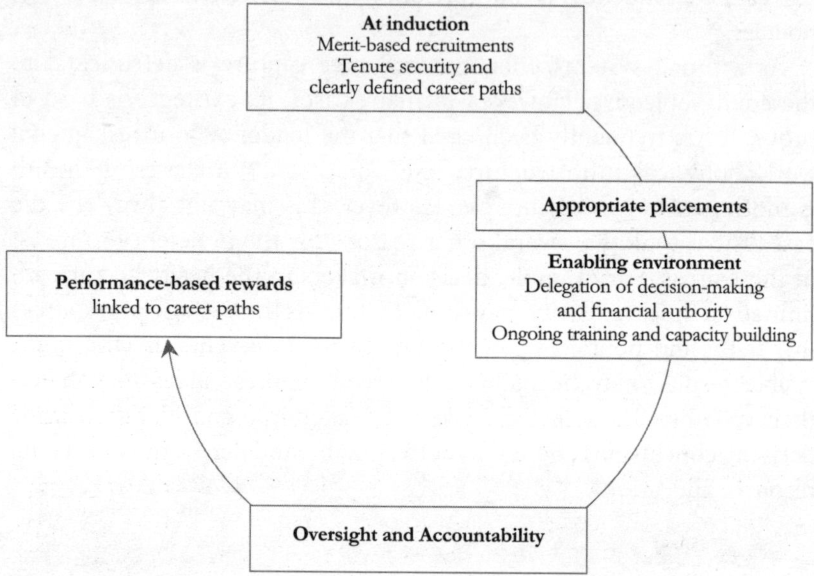

A number of problems are currently prevalent at every stage of the public management cycle in Pakistan. First, are issues of capacity, as have been described earlier under the section on *Setting strategic directions*. Issues of capacity stem from lack of core competencies and training. Majority of officers serving in the federal and provincial governments, who do not belong to any cadre or service, do not receive systematic training for upgrading their technical and managerial skills. This augments the capacity deficit, as a result of which, deployment often does not match needed skills. All these factors have a negative impact on the quality of governance.

Secondly, there is limited understanding of what human resource management entails. In the public sector, human resource management is generally considered as being synonymous with the creation of posts, placement of staff, and disciplinary action and is, as such, often used as a lever of power and patronage. Human resource planning usually does not appear to be a priority and human resource management, as a function, does not exist in most administrative domains in the public sector. Such an institutional outlook is particularly detrimental for ex-cadre administrators and senior managers, for whom there are no career paths and tenure security.

Thirdly, the environment is not conducive to fostering improvements in performance. The system does not reward high performers, in general. Rules and regulations governing administrative and financial prerogatives are overtly cumbersome and tend to centralize decision-making. There is limited autonomy of decision-making, even for trivial matters. For example, all transfers and postings—even for the lowest grades in the government system—are decided by the highest level of authority. This, coupled with limited conference of powers to take appropriate disciplinary action, is an impediment to ensuring compliance with rules and ethical standards. All these factors negatively influence performance.

Clarity in roles, responsibilities, and prerogatives is another factor that contributes to the creation of an enabling environment. Lack of clarity in this respect, particularly with reference to provincial district relationships, has additional negative implications for performance. This has been described in detail in the chapter on *Institutional Reform* under *Decentralization.*

In the fourth place, malpractices are well-institutionalized in human resource recruitments and placements, both in administrative positions as well as in the case of health service providers. With reference to recruitments, preferential treatment to well-connected individuals and unfair hiring practices are well-ingrained in the system. These are less frequent, where several levels of systems and procedures are in place, particularly in high-end clinical jobs such as in the case of specialist doctors. Here, peer oversight is a critical factor in ensuring some level of conformity with stipulated rules. However, despite this, there are many ways of bypassing procedures. For example, the timing of an advertisement for a key clinical job can be modified to suit particular individuals in terms of their completing a degree or fulfilling a particular job prerequisite. Similarly, the exact specifications and requirements of a job can be tampered with.

In case of higher administrative and non-clinical positions, cronyism in public sector appointments is well described. Misuse of public authority to influence hiring is also common in case of staff hiring for lower administrative positions. Here, competitive qualifications do not pose an impediment to selection. Additionally, informed peer oversight is minimal. In these settings, even when hiring is purportedly done through an open competitive process, sanction letters are often awarded directly from politically appointed representatives. All these malpractices in hiring and recruitments have negative implications for competency, capacity, performance, and staff morale.

Lastly, because of limited accountability and transparency, poor governance, and mismanagement, inefficiencies and corruption have become deeply institutionalized in the public management process. Poor management and lack of accountability exacerbate corruption, whereas on the other hand, there may be a disincentive for administrators to strengthen management and mainstream mechanisms that compel accountability. Both these factors complement each other in a vicious cycle. Limited accountability is the core determinant of this pattern. This gap exits both at the levels of performance accountability as well as financial accountability.

Limited accountability and transparency can manifest in a number of malpractices in the public management process. These can range from financial malpractices in contracting and procurements to malpractices in administrative and regulatory domains. Amongst other things, the latter can include collusion in granting permissions and malpractices at the level of monitoring to ensure compliance with stipulated standards in the domains of quality, price, and volume regulation. In such cases, commissions, bribes, and deliberate inattention to oversight are anecdotally reported to be endemic. Administrative corruption can also include the moral, procedural, and financial forms of malpractices where discretionary funds can be embezzled, inspectors may be deliberately inattentive to oversight, and providers can get by and moonlight in the private sector, pilfer state funds, and charge costs for services that are meant to be provided free of cost by the state.

Deliberate lack of oversight and inattention to mechanisms that compel accountability by senior public officials is most pronounced in the healthcare sector in the case of managerial reluctance to confront physicians in public hospitals on account of malpractices, which have been described in the chapter on *Service Delivery*. In the same chapter, a pattern of malpractice has been described under *Field delivery of services*, where lack of attention to oversight at the field level is the result of collusion, which enables pilfering of state resources and misdirecting of subsidies and services for private gains. Other forms of deliberate inattention to oversight in cases of human resource misconduct in the public administrative arena, delivery of publicly financed services, and regulation of private sector have also been well described and are addressed in various sections of this publication. All these factors act together to undermine performance, institutionalize malpractices within the system, and foster attitudinal maladies, thereby undermining the equity objective of health.

3.2.2.ii Parallel management system

As already stated, there are a number of critical weaknesses in Pakistan's public management system in the healthcare sector. Low incentives and lack of performance and financial accountability have led to institutionalization of a number of malpractices in the management of public resources. These have been referred to in various sections of this publication and can largely be categorized as: (i) malpractices in public procurements; (ii) abuse of regulatory powers and oversight prerogatives; and (iii) moral, procedural, and financial forms of corruption in service delivery and management of public resources. Anecdotal reports have described the existence of organized channels that allow engagement in such malpractices and enable sharing of pilfered resources in many institutional settings, particularly in health facilities and hospitals. The most illustrative example of this is the manner in which mark-ups are institutionally shared.

Markups or 'commissions' are commonly levied in the procurement process; vulnerable areas include procurement of medicines, related products and equipment, and service contracts. In such cases, common corrupt practices include collusion in the process of bidding, inappropriate incentives to influence the selection process, and deliberate inattention to the winning contractor's performance. The process can also involve overinvoicing and overpayment by agencies so that the margin can be shared back. In the case of medicines and equipment, procurement officers can also 'facilitate' purchase of sub-standard consignments or promote a quantitative compromise and pocket the difference in price.

In well-institutionalized arrangements, kickbacks and commissions are distributed according to predetermined percentages and formulae amongst those involved in the process. In many settings, the commission-based system is so well-institutionalized that a parallel system operates but in a much more coordinated manner than the one officially managing public resources. Commissions are usually channelled into a 'fund', which is managed and disbursed according to unwritten but clearly stipulated procedures. These funds are given different names in various facilities. The most popular connotation used is 'Kitty Fund'.

The Kitty Fund and its namesakes have several other sources of contribution in áddition to procurement-related commissions (Figure 11). In hospitals, funds generated from forged medico-legal cases, under-reported outpatient registrations, and a percentage of the salary of staff 'allowed' to be absent from duty are usually added to the fund. Another source of contribution is the reimbursement channel. A number of autonomous agencies in Pakistan provide health coverage to millions of individuals and their dependants by reimbursing predetermined health providers for services rendered and retail outlets for medication provided. In this model, autonomous agencies usually have contracts with retail stores, to whom they give supply orders against which regular payments are made. This system can be abused at various levels—by doctors charging a fee for writing fake prescriptions or by retailers charging a commission for processing them or buying the prescription from patients at a percentage of its cost. These funds are channelled either to a range of beneficiaries through the Kitty Fund according to predetermined percentages or are individually pocketed.

Another source of contribution to the Kitty Fund is the billing system. Commissions and percentages are sometimes charged by officers in the finance and account departments to process bills presented by suppliers. However, this is dependant on the integrity of the officers in charge because in the absence of their 'patronage,' these malpractices become very difficult. Commissions levied may or may not be diverted through Kitty Funds, as they can also end up in individual pockets. In addition to established percentages according to which funds are distributed from the Kitty Fund to a number of predetermined beneficiaries, the Kitty Fund is also used for emergency purposes such as paying off an unexpected auditor.

Devolution of the government system in 2001,[222,223] and the resulting administrative and political decentralization of powers has impacted the parallel management system in a 'novel' manner. The district administration has traditionally had a more institutionalized control over both the public management process as well as the parallel management system. However, after decentralization, the political administration was

Figure 11. Sources of contribution to the 'Kitty Fund' in health facilities

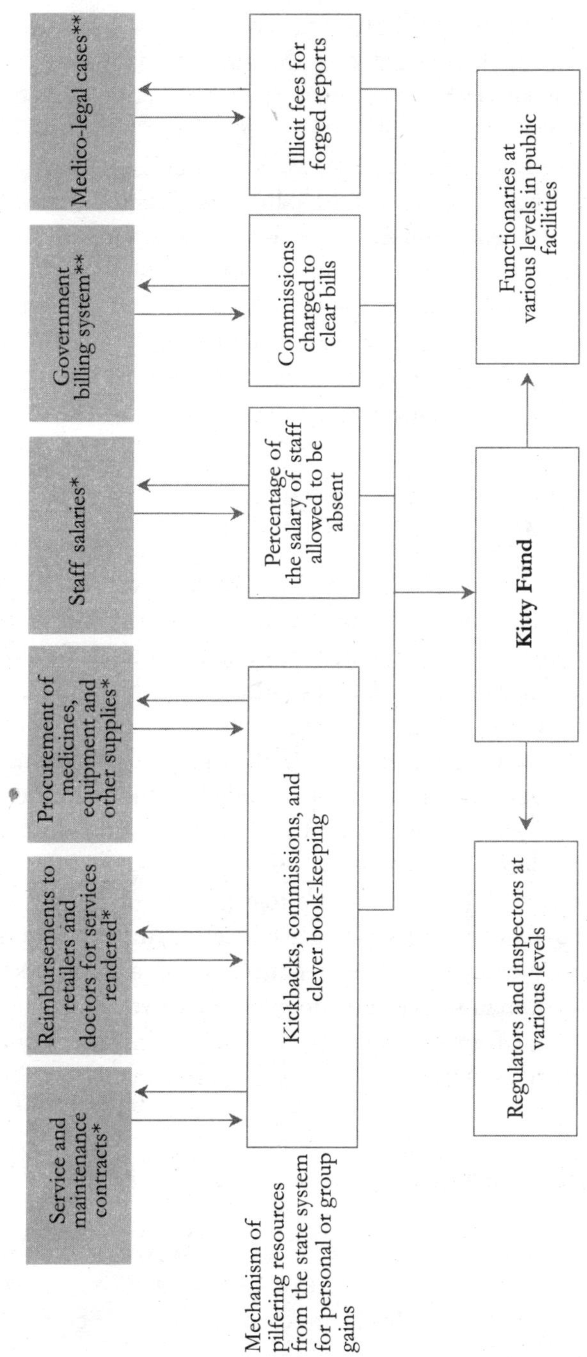

* Collusion in the use of state funds for personal gains
** Other means of illicit personal gains

quick to learn about the benefits of having access to such controls. This resulted in frequent turf battles between the district political and civil administration over procurement authority and contracting decisions.

It is difficult to prove the actual existence of a Kitty Fund and map its sources of contribution and dissemination channels in a particular setting because such funds do not leave a paper trail. There is, however, enough evidence of their existence to prioritize measures to break this vicious institutional cycle. Recommendations articulated in this publication aim to address these through a two-pronged approach—appropriate remuneration coupled with accountability on the one hand, and leveraging of technology as a deterrent against the current exploitation of manual record keeping, on the other.

3.2.3 Regulation

Regulation can be defined as an intervention initiated by the government to correct market failure. Conventionally, it refers to the use of state power to impose constraints on organizations and individuals through a range of legal instruments—laws, decrees, orders, administrative rules, and guidelines—issued by the government or non-governmental bodies to which the government has delegated regulatory powers. Incentives and behaviour change are generally not included in the definition of regulation. However, self-regulation and market regulation do factor these into consideration.

In the health sector, regulation can be relevant to quality, price, or numbers in the domain of services, medical education, human resource, food quality, and medicines and related technologies. Table 4 shows that for many of these domains, Pakistan does not have an effective and dedicated institutional framework in place, whereas in others, major gaps can be identified. A snapshot is provided of each area.

3.2.3.i Regulation of healthcare service delivery

Three regulatory considerations are relevant to private sector healthcare provision. These include authorization to establish facilities, ensuring compliance with quality standards, and output-based control of

Table 4. Health regulation in Pakistan

Areas of regulation	Responsible institution
Healthcare services in the private sector*	
Permission to establish facilities	No regulatory framework
Licensing quality standards	ibid
Control of service price	ibid
Accreditation	ibid
Medical education in the private sector	
Permission to establish facilities and numbers entering medical schools	Pakistan Medical and Dental Council
Licensing quality standards	ibid
Human resource in the private sector	
Licensing	Pakistan Medical and Dental Council; Pakistan Nursing Council; Pakistan Pharmacists Council
Pharmaceuticals	
Quality regulation	Ministry of Health
Price regulation	ibid
Intellectual Property Rights regulation	Not clearly defined at present
Medical technologies and equipment	
Quality regulation	No regulatory framework
Price regulation	ibid
Intellectual Property Rights regulation	ibid

* See explanation regarding provincial health regulatory authorities in the text

service prices. Two of the four provincial governments—NWFP and Balochistan—attempted to initiate regulation in these areas by establishing health regulatory authorities. However, both the institutions have not performed their mandated roles. Recently, efforts are underway to revitalize NWFP's health regulatory authority.

The significance of creating an appropriate regulatory framework for private sector healthcare provision in the country can hardly be overemphasized. An important caveat in this regard relates to limitations of the currently employed command and control style of regulation, which involves implementation of rules through administrative controls and enforcement of sanctions through onsite inspections, as this style of regulation is known to breed rent-seeking. Examples of malpractices outlined in the section on *Malpractices at the field level* in the chapter on *Service Delivery* are instructive in this regard. Regulation of private healthcare service provision should centre on introducing elements of market harnessing means of regulation, peer oversight, and self-regulation. With appropriate safeguards and transparent oversight, such regulatory frameworks can enable self-regulation of prices, quality as well as numbers. The manner in which such regulation needs to be mainstreamed in concert with service delivery reforms also has a bearing on institutional restructuring. This consideration has been discussed further in the chapter on *Institutional Reform*.

3.2.3.ii Regulation of health workforce and medical education

A number of professional organizations are currently mandated to regulate Pakistan's health workforce. Doctors and dentists are under the regulatory control of the Pakistan Medical and Dental Council (PMDC); human resource issues relevant to nurses are governed by the Pakistan Nursing Council; regulatory prerogatives of relevance to paramedics and pharmacists are delegated to relevant regulatory agencies, whereas practitioners of traditional medicine come under the purview of respective councils of *Tibb* and Homeopathy. In addition to professional licensing and recognition of training, these agencies are meant to grant permissions to establish training facilities of relevance to the related discipline, set standards and norms of individual and institutional behaviour, ensure compliance with standards, and stipulate the number of students entering relevant schools. In certain cases, regulatory agencies also exercise control over salary levels, remuneration, and other benefits.

The PMDC exercises oversight and control through peer regulation. This form of regulation generally holds merit because staff well qualified to assess performance is involved in regulation. However, peer regulation can also fall prey to 'regulatory capture,' which can result in it being self-serving and defending individual members. For instance, in PMDC's case, there has been a long-standing observation that the council does not adequately publicize malpractice cases and avoids taking due action against doctors who become party to promoting hospitality-based incentive-intense marketing practices. In addition, its relative silence on the issue of dual practice of public physicians is also a matter of concern. The selectivity of areas where professional associations choose to leverage their collective strength to voice their opinion raises additional apprehensions. Handing over of public hospitals to private medical schools without due regard to quality or need, unnecessary granting of permissions to upscale the number of students entering private medical schools and conferring undue recognition to schools that do not fulfil criteria can be regarded as manifestations of 'regulatory capture.'

Other than these long-standing and unresolved issues, the recent long-drawn scuffle over decision-making prerogatives between the PMDC and the Ministry of Health—one that has involved the Supreme Court's intervention on many occasions, provides insights into lack of clarity that state agencies have about regulatory independence. The PMDC is a body to which the government has delegated regulatory powers. It must empower it in that role without the need for complex hierarchical relationships. However, in order to serve this role well, the council must build safeguards against regulatory capture by establishing independent and impartial representation in governance, fostering an open information and disclosure policy, and creating effective and unpoliticized mechanisms of redress.

3.2.3.iii Regulation of food quality

Sanitary inspectors are meant to regulate food outlets and production facilities such as bakeries, meat shops and food vendors, factories, and hotels to ensure quality. As part of the scope of their work, they are meant to give advice on sanitary ethics, conduct inspections to ensure compliance with stipulated standards, and take punitive action in case of non-compliance. Because of inadequate remuneration, inspectors are forced to engage in bribes—a phenomenon some food manufacturers and retailers have a vested interest in promoting. In addition to isolated bribes, a monthly system of remuneration also exists to keep food inspectors at bay.

Aside from food and sanitary inspectors, a range of other regulatory institutional entities also subsist on this pattern. In addition, the intransigency with which the judicial system processes and prosecutes such cases is a major deterrent to institutionalizing accountability and justice.

All these examples testify the existence of several regulatory challenges within the health sector. These principally stem from the command and control style of regulation by low paid inspectors and regulators who operate in a public regulatory system where there are many opportunities for exploitation and limited accountability for deliberate inattention to mechanisms that compel accountability. A number of measures recommended in the sections on *Policy* and *Institutional Reform* in the chapter on *Reform within the Healthcare Sector* are important in addressing these issues. These include institutionalizing integrity in public service, mainstreaming market-harnessing means of regulation, and separating the policy-making, implementation, and regulatory functions within the government system. According to the directions of institutional reform proposed in this publication, *policy-making* should be entrusted to state agencies, *implementation* should be assigned to attached but functionally autonomous agencies whereas *regulatory* functions should be dedicated to fully-autonomous independent regulatory agencies. In relation to the latter, an important caveat is the level of autonomy. Autonomy should be fully autonomous in the administrative and financial sense, albeit with appropriate oversight. The governance of autonomous institutions should be independent, representative, unbiased, and technically sound and the chain of accountability should obviate commandeering by vested interest groups. Regulatory agencies have to be mandated and empowered so that they do not end up performing the clearing-house function, as some currently do. Additionally, they should be adequately resourced by the state so that there is no conflict of interest, as is presently the case with some regulatory agencies, which are meant to generate their own revenues.[224]

Regulation of medicines has been discussed in the chapter on *Medicines and Related Products.*

3.3 Reforming health governance

Reform of health governance must be capable of addressing the broad range of issues discussed in this chapter under *Setting Strategic Directions, Implementation and Oversight and Regulation.*

Firstly, an overarching issue is to foster transparency in governance. The chapter section on *Structural Reform of the State and Health* alludes to the policy and institutional imperatives, broader measures, and sectoral approaches in public sector reform, which have a bearing on addressing malpractices and outlines the role of actors outside of the healthcare sector in this regard. Technocratic reform in the civil service domain and sectoral reform in public financial management, procurement, and audit are important areas for systemic reform, which can deeply impact health governance. It is also important to proactively advocate for structural changes within the broader state system in order to mainstream overall transparency in governance. Reform of political institutions and the judiciary, civil society oversight, freedom of information, open media, avenues for seeking consumer redress and economic reforms that weaken the concentration of organized economic vested interest assume significance in this regard.

Secondly, reform of the public management process is critical. The chapters on *Institutional Reform* and *Human Resource* present options to address several human resource issues currently prevalent in the public management process—absence of career structures and tenure security for ex-cadre administrators, malpractices in recruitment, discrepancies in placement, the deployment-capacity mismatch, limited opportunities for capacity building and an environment that does not foster improvements in performance. In order to strengthen the public management process and thereby enhance performance of state functionaries and foster a result- and accountability-based culture, attention will have to focus both on the *creation of an enabling milieu*—market compatible incentives, building capacity and decentralizing decision-making and fiscal controls—as well as *enhancing accountability.*

In the third place, the section on *Institutional Reform* in the chapter on *Reform within the Health System* discusses several institutional considerations, which underpin reform of governance. Reform of the Ministry of Health and the provincial departments of health—agencies with a stewardship role—should focus on capacity building in order to enable them to serve their normative and oversight roles better and reconfigure their capacities so that they can deliver on the Health for All premise, leveraging the strength of all actors within the health system.

Reform of governance is also deeply interwoven with transparency and effectiveness of regulatory arrangements and the manner in which regulation is held at an independent arms length relationship from policy-making and implementation roles in state-mandated agencies. Restructuring of state and quasi-state organizational entities should clearly assign functions of policy-making, regulation, and implementation to appropriate state and quasi-state agencies and must grant administrative and financial autonomy in line with the principles of subsidiarity. Issues related to decentralization of the government system and the resulting unattended ambiguities, which undermine functioning of the local government system, also merit close consideration. In addition, institutional reform should focus on fostering greater inter-sectoral coordination and synergizing health and population, which exist as separating institutional entities in the country. These issues have been discussed in the chapter section on *Institutional Reform*.

Lastly, it is important to inculcate democratic behaviour at the individual and institutional levels in governance and institutionalize democratic values of liberty, equality, freedom, and rights as an institutional norm. Without these attributes, isolated technocratic changes at the governance level will have limited impact.

Chapter 4

Health Financing

The mode of health financing is one of the major factors determining both the configuration as well as the performance of a health system. Any envisaged health systems reform can, therefore, use changes in the modes of health financing as an entry point to reforming the entire system. The major disparity in health financing in Pakistan, as in many other developing countries, relates to the predominance of private means of financing—out-of-pocket payments—as opposed to public means of financing healthcare. The latter, which are more desirable, include revenues and pooling. This chapter attempts to approach the issue by outlining current gaps and opportunities under the three broad health financing categories of *collection*, *pooling* and *purchasing* and suggests a way forward to reform the current health financing model in Pakistan. In doing so, the envisaged impact of the recent global and domestic economic downturn on availability of resources has been given due consideration.

4.1 Pakistan's health financing landscape

A description of Pakistan's health systems is given in chapter 1. For greater clarity in comprehending Pakistan's health financing landscape, it is recommended that this section be read in conjunction with the overview of health systems articulated therein. The description coins some institutions and health actors as systems in their own right, given their *vertical* orientation. These include the Armed Forces health system, the Fauji Foundation system and the Employees Social Security Institute (ESSI), each of which has mutually exclusive service delivery infrastructure and human resource and governance arrangements. Together, they serve 22.28 million employees and their dependants (Table 6). The Armed Forces health system is financed through tax revenues, the Fauji Foundation system through profits from the organization's commercial activities, which are predetermined for social protection, and the ESSI through compulsory social security contributions made by employers.

Other systems shown in Figure 4 (chapter 2) access a mix of public and private service providers for care and have, therefore, been described as being *horizontal*. General revenues finance healthcare for government employees whereas autonomous organizations and corporate entities provide health coverage to their employees and their dependants by pooling for risk either through insurance or by reimbursing providers. The percentage of the population these systems cover and the total health expenditure they account for is presented in Tables 5a and 6. These data show that 26.62 per cent of the country's population is covered—at least partially—for healthcare costs. However, most people access care through out-of-pocket payments made directly to private providers at the point of care. An estimated 73.38 per cent of the population—representing 115.04 million individuals—is not fully covered for healthcare costs (Table 6).[225]

4.2 Collection

There are principally six modes of collection within the country: public revenues, out-of-pocket payments, donor contributions, employers' contributions, philanthropy, and commercial profits predetermined for social protection. Out-of-pocket payments are the major mode of collection, as they constitute 57.33 per cent of the total spending on health. This is followed by revenues, which account for 33.32 per cent. Employers' contributions, donors, commercial profits and philanthropy contribute 5.07 per cent, 1.72 per cent, 1.64 per cent, and 0.92 per cent, respectively (Table 7).

4.2.1 General revenue pool

Public revenue mobilization in Pakistan is low by international standards. Most of the revenue is generated at the federal level and is distributed to the federal government and the provinces by the National Finance

Table 5a. Sources of health financing in Pakistan

	Annual health expenditures in Pak. Rs. and (US $)[Δ] in million		Percentage of total health expenditure
Public sources	**Total**		
1. Revenues			
A. Federal government			
Health and other*[1]	12,167.00 (202.78)		5.86
Population welfare*[1]	4,241.00 (70.68)		2.04
Education*[1]	5.00 (0.08)		0.002
Military health expenditure*•[1]	7,452.00 (124.20)		3.59
Government employees*•[2]‡	615.10 (10.25)		0.30
State functionaries in judiciary and legislature*•[2]‡	59.84 (1.00)		0.03
	24,539.94 (409.00)		**11.83**
B. Provincial government			
Health and other*[1]	15,089.00 (251.48)		7.27
Population welfare*[1]	2,181.00 (36.35)		1.05
Education*[1]	1,737.00 (28.95)		0.84
Government employees*•[2]‡	9,880.60 (164.68)		4.76
State functionaries in judiciary and legislature*•[2]‡	531.99 (8.87)		0.26
	29,419.59 (490.33)		**14.18**
C. District bodies			
District governments*[1]	14,080.00 (234.67)		6.79
Cantonment boards*[1]	167.00 (2.78)		0.08
	14,247.00 (237.45)		**6.87**
D. Government's safety nets*[3]‡	925.91 (15.43)		0.45
		69,132.44 (1,152.21)	**33.32**
2. Publicly mandated private means			
Autonomous bodies†•[4]‡	5,170.80 (86.18)		2.49
Employees Social Security Institute*•[1]	2,052.00 (34.20)		0.99
Fauji Foundation System*•[5]‡	3,401.02 (56.68)		1.64
		10,623.82 (177.06)	**5.12**
3. Official donor assistance*[1]		**3,565.00 (59.42)**	**1.72**
Total for public sources		**83,321.26 (1,388.69)**	**40.16**

Continued...

Table 5a. Continued...

	Annual health expenditure in Pak. Rs. and (US $)$^{\Delta}$ in million		Percentage of total health expenditure
Private Sources			
1. Private sources of pooling			
Private employers[†•6]	3,300.00 (55.00)		1.59
Philanthropy[†7]	1,910.32 (31.84)		0.92
		5,210.32 (86.84)	**2.51**
2. Out of pocket payments*[1,8]		**118,952.00 (1,982.53)**	**57.33**
Total for private sources		**124,162.32 (2,069.37)**	**59.84**
Grand Total		**Rs. 207,483.58 $ (3,458.06)**	**100.00**

* Officially reported figures

† Estimations, with details explained in the relevant footnote

‡ Data adjusted for inflation rate (based on CPI) with reference to year 2005/06

Δ US $ exchange rate Pak. Rs. 60 (average for the year 2005/06)

◆ Employers cover health expenses of employees and their dependants

1. National Health Accounts for 2005-06; Statistics Division, Federal Bureau of Statistics, 2009. Accessible at http://www.statpak.gov.pk/depts/fbs/publications/national_health_account2005_06/National_Health_Accounts.pdf
2. Communications no: F.2(3)PF.I/2005-457 dated 27 March 2008 from the Ministry of Finance; Government of Pakistan. The figures shown account for expenses that are reimbursed and are additional to the free care provided at government hospitals.
3. The government's safety net arrangements include Zakat (Muslim charity) and Bait-ul-Mal (cash transfer programme). The amount shown represents health-specific allocations as evidenced by respective annual reports: (i) Final utilization report of Zakat Fund for the year 2006/07, Ministry of Religious Affairs, Government of Pakistan; and (ii) Pakistan Bait-ul-Mal Annual Report 2005/06, Ministry of Social Welfare and Special Education, Government of Pakistan. For this analysis, the government's contributions in both these areas have been regarded as falling within the rubric of safety net. However, it is recognized that by definition, other sources of financing which have been listed under publicly-mandated private means also fall within the same area.
4. Actual reported data on health expenditure for 77.5 per cent of the employees of federal autonomous agencies has been provided by the Ministry of Finance, Government of Pakistan, vide their communication no: No 1 (1)-CF.II/2008-part/571 dated 30 April 2008. Per capita estimates derived have been extrapolated to the rest of the 22.5 per cent of the federal employees and their dependants.
5. Verbal communication with Fauji Foundation, Pakistan; September 2008.
6. According to marketing surveillance estimates, private health insurance covers 1,000,000 individuals in Pakistan; their premium contributions are estimated at Rs. 3300 (US $55) per capita, per annum (personal communication with Harris Nazir, Deputy General Manager, Allianz EFU Health Insurance Limited, Karachi, Pakistan: September 2008).
7. Non-profit organizations in the health sector registered with the Pakistan Centre for Philanthropy report their funding sources (http://www.pcp.org.pk/resources.html) under three heads: self-generated income and national and international grants/donations. International and national grants were taken into account. Private philanthropic contributions could not be included as described in the text.
8. Annual per-capita health expenditures have been derived from monthly per-capita health expenditures reported in the Pakistan Social and Living Standards Measurement survey report, 2005/06. These data were used in the National Health Accounts 2005/06.

Table 5b. Health expenditure by the public and private sectors

	Yearly expenditure in Pak. Rs. and (US $) in million	Yearly per capita expenditure in Pak. Rs. and (US $)	Percentage of GDP[Δ]
Public sources*	83,321.26 (1,388.69)	531.49 (8.86)	1.16
Private sources**	124,162.32 (2,069.37)	792.00 (13.20)	1.73
Total	207,483.58 (3,458.06)	1323.49 (22.06)	2.90

* Public sources include contributions from federal and provincial governments, district bodies, safety nets, publicly mandated private measures, and official donor assistance.
** Private sources include pooling from private employers, philanthropy and out of pocket payments.
Δ GDP(fc) = Pak. Rs. 7,158,527 million (Economic Survey 2005/06)

Commission according to a formula, which primarily takes provincial population estimates into account. Within provinces, the Provincial Finance Commissions decide on allocation of funds to districts, based on estimates derived by the districts themselves. It is at the discretion of the district to internally allocate funds within various departments. The provincial governments do not presently have the leverage to stipulate earmarking of a certain percentage of general revenues to areas such as health, which usually feature low on the list of priorities within districts. The districts also have an additional line of fund transfer from the federal government, outside of the provincial district accounting channels. These are tight grants earmarked for implementing national public health programmes described in the chapter on *Service Delivery*. On-budget donor resources are also sometimes channelled in this manner.

Allocations for health from the general revenue pool are not fully integrated at the federal, provincial, and district levels, nor do they explicitly support common health objectives. Often, expenditure patterns do not follow stated priorities in overarching instruments such as the Poverty Reduction Strategy Paper (PRSP). In addition, there are no mechanisms in place to evaluate the impact of given allocations on outcomes vis-à-vis the equity objective. It is, therefore, important to develop an overarching mechanism to ensure that federal, provincial, and district allocations jointly contribute to achieving a consistent and coherent set of nationally agreed objectives in line with stated priorities. The federal government should work with the provinces and districts to develop mechanisms so that a percentage of the development expenditure in the districts is spent on the delivery of health. In addition, it should

Table 6. Segments of the population receiving comprehensive/partial financial coverage for health in Pakistan

		Annual health expenditure in Pak. Rs. and (US $)[Δ] in million	Total number of beneficiaries/ employees and their dependants covered (in million)	Health expenditure per person in Pak. Rs. and (US $)[Δ]	Percentage of the total population** of Pakistan covered
Formally employed sector					
A	Government*				
	Federal government	615.10 (10.25)	3.22	190.93 (3.18)	2.06
	Provincial government	9,880.60 (164.68)	11.78	838.60 (13.98)	7.52
B	State functionaries in the judiciary and legislature*				
	Federal level	59.84 (1.00)	0.04	1,413.71 (23.56)	0.03
	Provincial level	531.99 (8.87)	0.18	3,029.06 (50.48)	0.11
C	Armed forces	7,452.00 (124.20)	6.29	1,184.55 (19.74)	4.01
D	Publicly mandated private means				
	Autonomous bodies	5,170.80 (86.18)	2.73	1,894.44 (31.57)	1.74
	Employees Social Security Institute	2,052.00 (34.20)	6.89	297.90 (4.97)	4.39
	Fauji Foundation system	3,401.02 (56.68)	9.10	373.74 (6.23)	5.80
E	Private employers	3,300.00 (55.00)	1.00	3,305.65 (55.09)	0.64
Total		**32,463.35 (541.06)**	**41.23**	**787.39 (13.12)**	**26.30**
Informally employed sector					
	Government's safety nets	925.91 (15.43)	0.50	1,852.49 (30.87)	0.32
Total		**925.91 (15.43)**	**0.50**	**1,852.19 (30.87)**	**0.32**
Grand Total		**33,389.26 (556.49)**	**41.73**	**800.15 (13.34)**	**26.62**

* The figures shown account only for reimbursements for medical care costs, which are additional to free care at government facilities

** Total population: 156.77 million for the year 2005/6 (Source: Economic Survey 2006-07); Δ US $ exchange rate Pak. Rs. 60 (average for the year 2005/06)

Table 7. Sources of collection

		Percentage of contributions	
Revenues	Federal government	11.83	
	Provincial government	14.18	
	District bodies	6.87	
	Government's safety nets	0.45	
			33.32
Employers	Autonomous bodies	2.49	
	ESSI	0.99	
	Private employers	1.59	**5.07**
Donors			**1.72**
Commercial profits			**1.64**
Philanthropy			**0.92**
Out of pocket payments			**57.33**
			100.00

also use fiscal tools as an incentive to encourage the provinces and districts to enhance health allocations using performance-based criteria as a pre-conditionality and assist with capacity building in this regard.

Estimates for the year 2005/06 show that the public sector currently spends 1.16 per cent of the GDP on health. Overall, 2.90 per cent of the GDP was spent on health, with the private sector contributing the remainder (Table 5b). About 33.32 per cent of the total health expenditure for the year 2005/06 was funded from the general revenue pool. The total per capita health expenditure was estimated to be Rs. 1,323.49 (US $22.06). Of this, 40.16 per cent was contributed by the public sector and the rest by the private sector. These data underscore the need to allocate a higher share of existing revenues for health. The idea is to ensure funding for basic essential health services through the general pool of revenue. These services can be provided to citizens, both through a revitalized government Primary Health Care (PHC) system as well as by harnessing the outreach of private providers as has been described in the chapter on *Service Delivery*. The draft of the National Health Policy 2009, outlines the construct of a package, which is perceived as being essential, but has not estimated the cost if its delivery. The cost of a fully funded government system in Pakistan was previously estimated at US $21.12 per capita, per annum for one province (NWFP).[226] Other countries have also developed such packages at lower costs (US $14–17),[227,228] compared to the WHO-recommended US $34.[229] Building further on these experiences, the package of basic essential health services needs to be honed further and its cost estimated. The government should then review the Fiscal Responsibility and Debt Limitation Act 2005 and stipulate incremental increases in revenue allocations to a level where the delivery of basic essential services becomes possible.[230]

Several considerations merit attention while advocating for *enhancing revenue allocations for health.* First, it is acknowledged that taxation demands an extensive tax collection capacity and is possible largely in formal economies, whereas in Pakistan, the informal sector of the economy is predominant. Less than 1 per cent of Pakistan's population is registered as direct taxpayers. It is a challenge to optimize tax collection when the tax base is so small and when the informal economy is predominant.

The second important factor relates to the recent global and domestic economic downturn. Lack of integration of Pakistan's financial markets with international markets had precluded earlier importation of the crisis into Pakistan, as it did in other countries of East Asia, where financial markets are well integrated with the global financial system. This notwithstanding, the synergistic effect of other factors—poor governance, political instability, ongoing conflict, and the economic impact emanating from the crisis in international commodity markets—led to Pakistan's domestic economic meltdown from 2007 onwards. Although the recent injection of IMF's rescue resources and commitments of bilateral assistance are encouraging, they do not provide sustainable solutions for macroeconomic recovery and cannot create the direly needed fiscal space.

After the largest ever cuts in Public Sector Development Programme (PSDP) budgets in 2008/09,[231] the government has adopted an expansionary fiscal policy in the 2009/10 budget.[232] However, significant reliance on development assistance to fund the social sectors makes this an unviable and unsustainable approach. Although the United States has made an exception by increasing—rather than decreasing—bilateral assistance to Pakistan in this financially constrained milieu,[233] there are no indications that trends in overall development assistance will be likewise. All these factors indicate that fiscal space constraints will continue to prevail. Lessons from a review of events in history show that a financial crisis can actually galvanize political commitment for sustained social transformation because of its dire social impact. The

Great Depression of the 1930s and the subsequent evolution of social security in the United States and the establishment of the National Health Service in the United Kingdom after the Second World War are cases in point. The government of Pakistan can, therefore, use the financial crisis as an opportunity to enhance public commitment for health and other social sectors, and more broadly, galvanize a social transformation in the country.

Fiscal space constraints in relation to the PSDP and development assistance reiterate the need to explore innovative means of health financing in Pakistan. There are many examples from around the world, where innovative strategies have enabled the mobilization of additional resources and have created incentives for allocation in specific areas. For example, the International Finance Facility for immunization (IFFim) leverages pledges of governments' future donations for upfront cash on financial market bonds to support GAVI immunization programmes. In the Debt2Health initiative, a creditor—be it a donor government or a private company—relinquishes the right to partial repayment of previous loans on the condition that the beneficiary recipient country invests the freed-up resources in approved programmes of the Global Fund to Fight AIDS, Tuberculosis and Malaria (GFATM). In addition, prize funding mechanisms have been established as an additional incentive for Research and Development (R&D), and advance market commitments are being used to create a market sufficiently large and credible to stimulate private R&D and manufacturing and accelerate vaccine introduction in developing countries. There are also many examples from around the world, where earmarked taxes are being levied to support health—tobacco taxes have supported tobacco control efforts in many countries and recently UNITAID is being funded by an airline tax introduced in 27 countries. Other ideas have also been presented by the high-level Task Force on Innovative International Financing for Health Systems established in the context of the International Health partnership.[234]

Pakistan must carefully explore the potential within innovative approaches to raise resources and create incentives for their appropriation, where needed. Some headway has been made with the signing of the debt swap for €40 million with Germany and GFATM under the umbrella of the Debt2Health initiative.[235] However, many of the country's previous attempts at innovative financing have not been successful because of limited commitment within the system to target generated resources for intended purposes. The Ministry of Health has been imposing a percentage levy as tax on the net profits of pharmaceutical companies in Pakistan for years and the education sector has an earmarked tax called *Iqra*. However, the impact of these on financing arrangements has not been evident. These considerations should carefully be brought to bear in any future attempt at mainstreaming innovative financing for health. However, the question of whether a specific government resource can be earmarked for health—e.g., a health tax—should be very carefully considered in an environment where ear-marking of specific resources can undermine the commitment to funding from the general revenue pool.

Fiscal space constraints also draw attention to the poor correlation between total spending and health outcomes. Therefore, efforts to enhance allocations for health should be matched with initiatives to *improve returns on spending.* This can be done in many ways. Foremost is the need to improve fund utilization. The allocation-versus-expenditure lag in health has been well-described, although it has narrowed down in recent years.[236] Many factors negatively impact the ability to expend; these include excessive centralization of operational decision-making, onerous financial and administrative procedures, lack of accountability of decision-making delays, and limited capacity to plan and implement. An allied issue relates to *quality of expenditures*—tracking of budgetary fund flows in the public sector shows a predominance of expenditures in the month of May and June before the financial year ends, with non development budgets predominating. Therefore, alongside budgetary increases, it is critical to set aside dedicated funds for reforms that address fund utilization bottlenecks and focus on improving the quality of expenditure. It is also crucial to reduce the impact of inefficiencies, both at the level of allocation, which result in suboptimal allocation of available resources, as well as at the technical level to reduce inefficiencies in relation to the monies invested in programmes. This can be done through rationalization of transaction costs, improved integration of programmes, and better alignment of aid with national financing strategies, as outlined in the Paris Declaration on Aid Effectiveness, to which Pakistan is a signatory.

In terms of *returns on investments,* the effect of corruption on compromising public investments in a highly-constrained environment

must be taken into account. *Leakage of funds* from the system is an outcome of various forms of corruption, as has been alluded to throughout this publication. These occur because of poorly managed expenditure systems and poor fiscal controls over flow of public resources. Improving governance is critical to addressing these issues. From a budgetary standpoint, however, attention to certain areas can give quick dividends. For example, the use of technology and setting up of electronic public expenditure tracking systems and electronic equipment and supply inventories can help track leakages from the system, and a nationwide database for matching staff and wage payments can maintain up to date personal records and assist in eliminating abuses such as payments to ghost workers. Budgetary allocations should, therefore, leverage technology to enhance efficiency and promote greater transparency in the health system.

Alongside increase in allocations, *equitable allocation of revenue* should also be promoted to ensure that a wider faction of the population benefits from higher public expenditure. Here, it must be noted that 26.81 per cent of the total revenue allocation reflected in Table 5a, is allocated for 13.72 per cent of the population, which consists of government employees, members of the judiciary and legislature, and employees of the armed forces (Table 6). Allocations reflected in Table 5a are additionally underestimations since a proportion of the development budget is also allocated for government hospitals where 'entitled patients'—essentially federal and provincial government servants—receive free care. Thus, the total health expenditure per capita, in the case of employees in the afore-stated categories, is over and above the stated range (Table 6). Even if that is not taken into consideration, present estimates show that the government's per capita expenditure on health for this segment of the population, in most categories is higher than what it spends on the remaining 86.28 per cent of the population—per capita revenue expenditure on health for 135.26 million individuals is around Pak. Rs. 374.05 (US $6.23 per capita). These data highlight inequitable distribution of revenue allocations in the health sector. The idea here is not to discredit the approach to higher health expenditure for those in the service of the state, but to argue the case for providing similar coverage to all individuals in the country.

A few considerations merit attention with reference to the *distribution of financial resources* within the healthcare system. These include the distribution of resources within public health programmes and between the curative and preventive streams of work. With reference to the former, data from the Pakistan Demographic Surveys shows that the percentage of deaths attributed to Non-Communicable Diseases (NCDs) has increased from 34.1 per cent in 1992 to 59.99 per cent in 2005.[237] This trend is also supported by data from earlier burden-of-disease studies within the country.[238] However, resource allocations within public health in Pakistan do not take cognizance of the high burden of NCDs. This is evidenced by a comparison of the percentage attribution to each cause of death with preventive programme resource allocations in respective domains—a disparity that needs to be addressed (Figure 12). It is often argued that since NCDs are not included in the MDGs—the MDGs form the basis of Pakistan's health sector priorities—they do not qualify to be included in mainstream planning. Within this context, it must be appreciated that Goal 6 of the MDGs refers to 'other diseases' on the premise that countries would have the indigenous capacity to determine what constitutes a locally suited priority. Non-communicable diseases should clearly be a public health priority in Pakistan, given that they kill more people than malaria, tuberculosis and HIV and AIDS combined.

Figure 12. Percentage attribution to cause of death compared with resource allocations to respective preventive programmes

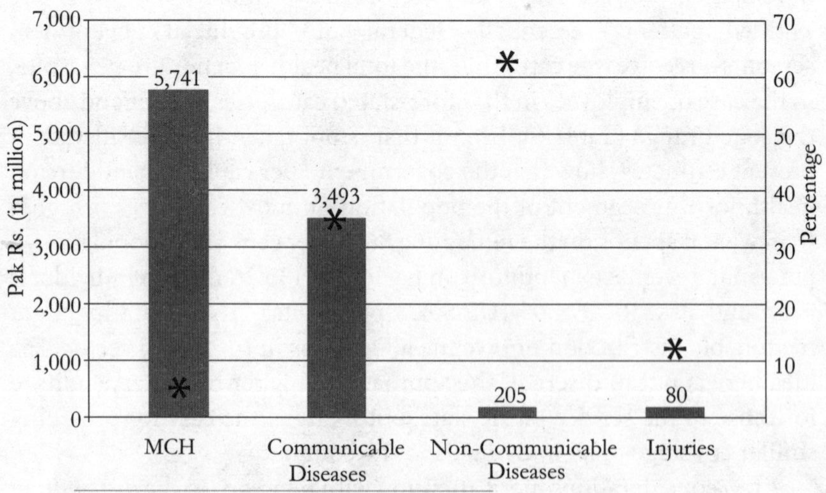

With reference to distribution of financial resources between the preventive and curative streams, balance dictates that whereas prevention and health promotion need to be prioritized and delivered as a public good, there is also valid justification for investing in hospitals, given that if left to the private market, curative care, being cost-intensive and rival in consumption, would be excludable for the poor. It is, therefore, important to ensure that state funds are used through appropriate waiver and exemption systems to ensure that the poor are not excluded from care provided in public hospitals, where user charges are usually levied.

4.2.2 Development assistance

Data relevant to donor contributions reflected in Table 5a, which were used to calculate health expenditures, have been reported from official sources—National Health Accounts, for the year 2005/06.[239] Based on this, donor contributions account for 1.72 per cent of the total health expenditure. However, in reality, these contributions are larger as the figure listed under the category 'donors' in Table 5a refers only to off-budget donor contributions. An attempt has, therefore, been made to examine the actual volume of donor contributions.

Calculating yearly contributions proved difficult because of a number of factors. A range of multilateral and bilateral donors, the UN system, and global health initiatives are currently contributing fiscal and in kind resources to assist with healthcare delivery in Pakistan. All these development agencies have projects of varying durations in different cycles. Resources are released at different times and archiving of details relevant to allocation, disbursement and expenditure in government and donors systems is often incomplete or inaccessible and sometimes, non-concordant. Furthermore, part of the allocation is embedded in government budgets and is hence even more difficult to track. In order to obviate some of these issues, yearly estimates have been computed by triangulating information from various sources—government of Pakistan's evolving Donor Assistance Database and information on disbursements received directly from some development partners.[240]

Table 8 summarizes yearly estimates of development assistance. Estimations from the information posted on the Development Assistance Database show that donors allocate 62.10 per cent of their

Table 8. Estimated yearly contributions to the health sector by development agencies in Pak. Rs. and (US$)$^{\Delta}$ in million

Donors	Maternal and child health	Training and advocacy	Infectious disease control	Medical services and PHC	Population welfare	Health information system	Non-Communicable diseases	Total
ADB*	348.10 (5.80)	-	-	-	-	-	-	348.10 (5.80)
CIDA*	50.26 (0.84)	1.95 (0.03)	61.40 (1.02)	1.46 (0.02)	-	-	-	115.07 (1.92)
DFID*	-	135.47 (2.26)	262.33 (4.37)	777.88 (12.96)	107.93 (1.80)	104.64 (1.74)	-	1,388.26 (23.14)
UNAIDS*	-	-	15.18 (0.25)	9.90 (0.16)	-	-	-	25.08 (0.42)
UNDP*	-	-	-	7.68 (0.13)	-	-	-	7.68 (0.13)
UNFPA*	40.71 (0.68)	32.02 (0.53)	-	31.15 (0.52)	-	-	-	103.89 (1.73)
UNICEF*	584.05 (9.73)	-	-	-	-	-	-	584.05 (9.73)
USAID*	420.34 (7.01)	-	212.52 (3.54)	1,595.48 (26.59)	471.65 (7.86)	79.46 (1.32)	-	2,779.46 (46.32)
World Bank*	-	-	257.38 (4.29)	2,069.85 (34.50)	-	-	-	2,327.23 (38.79)
WHO**	-	-	23.71 (0.40)	1.27 (0.02)	-	0.35 (0.01)	0.19 (0.003)	25.52 (0.43)
GAVI**	2,429.09 (40.48)	-	-	-	-	-	-	2,429.09 (40.48)
GFATM**	-	-	369.56 (6.16)	-	-	-	-	369.56 (6.16)
GTZ**	-	18.44 (0.31)	18.67 (0.31)	32.25 (0.54)	-	-	-	69.35 (1.16)
Packard Foundation**	-	54.69 (0.91)	-	-	112.20 (1.87)	-	-	166.89 (2.78)
Total	3,872.56 (64.54)	242.56 (4.04)	1,220.75 (20.35)	4,526.93 (75.45)	691.78 (11.53)	184.45 (3.07)	0.19 (0.003)	10,739.23 (178.99)

* Data from the Donor Assistance Database (http://www.dadpak.org/; accessed 21 May 2008, 12:50 pm). The amount reflected shows yearly disbursements under a set of seven programme categories. The amount was calculated by dividing cumulative disbursements for projects in each programme area by the number of years spanning the projects' duration. According to this information, 38 per cent of donor contributions are off-budget, whereas the remainder 62 per cent are on-budget.

** Data received from respective sources

Δ US $ exchange rate Pak. Rs. 60 (average for the year 2005/06) total allocations on budget. By extrapolating this percentage to the computations reflected in Table 5a, it appears that donors contribute an additional 3.21 per cent to total health expenditure for the year 2005/06. Collectively, this takes their estimated contribution to 4.93 per cent of the total health expenditure.

Development assistance has the potential to impact policies, governance structures, and planning instruments in Pakistan, not only by virtue of its size and the conditionalities it can stipulate as a precondition for funding, but also because of limited capacity within the state system, which inadvertently makes space for policies to be donor-driven. Many factors, therefore, merit careful attention with respect to allocation of development assistance in Pakistan.

Firstly, there is a concern that the current geopolitical and security motivation for much of the aid coming to Pakistan may subordinate social sector objectives. There has traditionally been a very strong correlation between geopolitical motivations and the volume of development assistance channelled into Pakistan. Increase in development assistance in the decade of 1954–64 in concert with Pakistan's signing of mutual defence assistance agreements with the US in the Cold War era; in the 1980s in the wake of the Afghan war; post-9/11 for obvious reasons and the troughs in the pattern of aggregate allocations in the periods in-between, are illustrative in this regard. A historical review of development assistance in Pakistan shows that integration of foreign policy and development objectives has not yielded far-reaching development dividends in Pakistan, so far. Donors must, therefore, clearly separate objectives and develop broad-based channels of communication so that they can benefit from impartial inputs from a broad constituency of stakeholders, and analyze the implications of integrating foreign policy and development objectives in Pakistan's complex body politic. The cost of inattention to the latter can be enormous, given the country's precarious situation and the vulnerability of its population to exploitation as violence, terrorism, and conflict pervade the national milieu.

Secondly, there appears to be a heightened expectation with respect to the potential within development assistance to improve social sector outcomes, most recently in the wake of the pledges made by the Friends of Democratic Pakistan and the passage of the Kerry–Lugar Bill.[241,242] The latter has trebled US assistance to Pakistan over a five-year period. In this hype, it is often forgotten that the best way to improve development outcomes is through sustaining growth, increasing employment rate and per capita income, and addressing the core disparities of power, money, and resources. Although aid can lend a strong impetus to development if it is of significant volume and is effectively used, expectations about its impact must be kept at reasonable levels in a country as large as Pakistan, where aid is often grafted on local institutions without strengthening them from within.

Thirdly, even if we imagine that development depended critically on external resource transfers, there are many sources besides aid, which should additionally be leveraged. Debt forgiveness and wiping out external indebtedness, coupled with better market access, are the two most important approaches in this regard. It is important to explore the amount of tariffs donors collect vis-à-vis the money they provide in aid. Facilitation of trade by dismantling the barriers to exports from Pakistan can be more important than traditional development assistance. Similarly, it is important to promote ethical 'export' of human resource on the premise that such an approach can enable earning foreign remittances, albeit whilst concomitantly building country capacity to ensure that the critically needed workforce is retained in the country by implementing workforce retention policies. Donors can also help widen the definition of public goods by easing some of the impediments that are inadvertently placed on development such as through Intellectual Property Rights, particularly in the domain of medical products and technological solutions. Pakistan will have to be fully compliant with the patent regime under the stipulations of World Trade Organization Agreements and Pakistan's Patent Ordinance, in 2016, which is when these considerations will assume importance. Most importantly, strategic technical inputs, subsidies, and diplomatic and market interventions in many other areas can ensure energy, food, environmental, and water security—all of them critically needed as the backbone of development, with important links with the health sector.

Lastly, improvements are needed in the donor disbursement strategy. The aid architecture in Pakistan is becoming increasingly complicated, with a large number of organizations pursuing many objectives—sometimes with duplicative agendas. Over the years, donors have rallied around a number of approaches and channels of disbursement and have experimented with project assistance, programme assistance and budget support. Project assistance led to intra-sectoral imbalances, because of which the Sector Wise Approach was implemented—this conversely led to inter-sectoral imbalances. Programme assistance was seen as a way of mitigating this. It was envisaged that by agreeing on a set of criteria with the government and reimbursing them according to a predetermined percentage, as in the case of the Social Action Programme (SAP), these could be mitigated. The Social Action Programme dominated social sector planning in Pakistan and donor disbursement strategies in the 1990s, but could not lead to the desired impact. More recently, the tendency to give aid on budget is the third disbursement channel—an approach endorsed by the Paris Declaration and Accra Agenda. Centred on harmonizing and coordinating aid and pooling aid in support of a particular strategy led by the government, this was envisaged to strengthen country systems and minimize duplication and high transaction costs of multiple donor inputs. The Organization for Economic Cooperation and Development (OECD) conducted two rounds of monitoring in 2006 and 2008 to measure the impact of the Paris Principles.[243] Although Pakistan was not one of the countries surveyed, the key findings of the survey, which draw attention to systemic challenges undermining aid effectiveness, are relevant to Pakistan.

Donors will soon be experimenting with yet another approach to disbursement, as part of the new package of assistance, by creating a multi-donor trust fund. The approach has the potential to be useful if the fund parameters include a truly impartial, inclusive, and participatory governance arrangement, open disclosure policies, and third party audit. However, alongside that, many other measures must also be concomitantly undertaken. The government of Pakistan should strengthen its fiduciary systems, whereas donors must be sensitive to considerations of conditionality and ensure that aid does not undermine local accountability.

In view of the above considerations, a proactive country-specific effort should be made to ensure that development assistance is actually needed in the country, that it fulfils a strategic priority need, that it will predictably and reliably support country-led efforts, and that it will neither have any explicit or implicit harmful effects in the country over the long term nor undermine the sustainability of programmes. Donors must invest in health as an investment where equity is the endpoint. However, the ultimate objective of development assistance should be to channel predictable development assistance to help strengthen systems with a view to ultimately transition away from aid.

4.2.3 Out-of-pocket payments

Out-of-pocket payments reported in this publication have been based on National Health Accounts data reported recently by the Federal Bureau of Statistics (FBS).[244] Estimates have been derived from monthly health expenditures, as reported by the Pakistan Social and Living Standards Measurement (PSLM) survey. The methodology of this survey has been criticized for lack of robustness in relation to health expenditure. In order to obviate this, a module on health expenditure has recently been introduced into the Household Income and Expenditure Survey of FBS for the years 2007–08, with technical support from Heartfile and the World Bank. This is envisaged to yield validated data on expenditure patterns in various domains by 2010.

Segregating out-of-pocket household expenditure by disease categories is currently not possible. The need to do so becomes important in the context of the current neglect of NCDs, which are not considered as being within the remit of Pakistan's poverty reduction strategies, with reference to health. Non-communicable diseases are known to incur significant costs in care; they undermine the income-generating capability of households and can perpetuate an acute poverty crisis. These diseases have clearly emerged as major contributors to costs of care in a recent population-based cross-sectional survey and need to be included in the remit of poverty reduction instruments.[245]

4.2.4 Employers' contributions

In Pakistan, employers' contributions for healthcare financing come from three sources; the Employees Social Security Institute (ESSI), autonomous quasi-state organizations, and private employers. These are described in chapter 1 and data have been reflected in Table 7 in this chapter. Data relating to employees of autonomous organizations have been provided by the Ministry of Finance and are based on actual reporting whereas data relevant to ESSI are cited from a published source. Marketing surveillance data have been used for computing contributions made by private employers. This information has been triangulated with the number of employees in private organizations envisaged to comply with global employment practices in order to estimate expenditures on health by the private sector. Together, they account for 5.07 per cent of the total health expenditure and collectively cover 6.77 per cent of the country's population (Table 5a and 6).

4.2.5 Commercial profits predetermined for social protection

Pakistan has a novel source of fund collection to finance a vertically integrated social protection system for 9.1 million individuals—ex-military and their dependants. The system materialized out of the Post-War Services Reconstruction Fund in 1942. This fund was meant to be used for settling soldiers in civil life after the Second World War. Less than 20 per cent of the total funds collected at the end of the war were placed under the administrative control of a committee with representatives from the three military establishments of West Pakistan in 1947.

The endowment was used to establish the Fauji Group, which currently has a commercial and a welfare arm. The former consists of enterprises, the profits of which support the welfare arm through which welfare services are delivered to 5.8 per cent of the country's population at the lowest per capita estimated cost—nine times less than what the government pays as per capita cost to provide coverage to members of the judiciary and legislature (Table 6). Health expenditure of the Fauji Foundation system represents 1.64 per cent of the country's total health expenditure. The use of this endowment can be regarded as a commercially viable and socially responsible use of an investment, despite the criticism that the military has received for this pattern of fund use in recent years.[246]

4.2.6 Philanthropic contributions

According to data obtained from the Pakistan Centre for Philanthropy (PCP), philanthropic contributions account for approximately 0.92 per cent of the total health spending in Pakistan (Table 5a). Non-profit health organizations registered with PCP report their funding sources under three categories—self-generated income, national donations, and international grants. The sum of national and international grants has been taken into account while estimating this figure. However, the actual volume of philanthropy in Pakistan is difficult to gauge and has, in all probability, been underestimated in the stated figure because of limitations of these data to fully capture individual philanthropy. The total value of individual philanthropy—monetary giving, both *Zakat* and non-*Zakat*, in kind gifts, and value of time volunteered by residents and diaspora of the country—has been estimated at Pak. Rs. 70 billion (US $1.08 billion) yearly by a study in 1998.[247]

The potential to finance health through philanthropy has not been fully tapped in Pakistan. Limited attempts have been made in the past to develop efficient and transparent institutional mechanisms to collect and effectively target funds to those in need. Heartfile is in the process of establishing a Health Financing pilot project with a view to bridging this gap.[248] The pilot aims to develop a transparent and expeditious mechanism to protect the poor against catastrophic expenditures on health—the key out-of-pocket expenditures, with significant economic implications for impoverishment. Innovations in technology on the request processing side and in donation management constitute the major novelties of this project.

With respect to donation management, the capability to instruct age, gender, disease, and region-specific donations and the capability to be responsive to demands on a real time basis are envisaged to bring unprecedented benefits to the donor in determining the use of allocated funds. In addition, the system's ability to update donors about utilization of their funds on a micro-transaction basis is an additional innovative feature, which is envisaged to contribute both to transparency as well as efficiency. The system will also be able to categorize patients by the level of urgency of treatment required, financial need, and by evaluating health expenditures vis-à-vis disposable income. Through tracking and time stamping as inherent features, it will additionally allow assessment of workers' performance and hence help to institutionalize accountability. It is envisaged that these specifications will allow cost-effective targeting of resources through appropriate categorization of patients in need, ensure better visibility to donors, and promote human resource and organizational efficiency. All these attributes will help Heartfile augment the base of its resources to finance healthcare for those that run the risk of spending catastrophically on health.

4.3 Pooling

From data presented in the previous section of this chapter, it is evident that private sources of health financing (out-of-pocket payments) are more predominant in Pakistan compared to public sources of financing (revenues and pooling). Revenue allocations account for 33.32 per cent of total health expenditure whereas pooling as a means of health financing accounts for 7.63 per cent.[249] Together, public and private sources account for 40.16 per cent and 59.84 per cent of the health expenditure, respectively. This is paradoxical since public sources are a more desirable form of financing and need to be maximized and mainstreamed in the health system. The previous section of this chapter has made a case for enhancement of revenues to finance the delivery of basic essential health services. This section will explore the potential within pooling as another source of public financing to cover the costs of services falling outside of the basic essential health service category.

Pooling is a mechanism to ensure that citizens do not have to pay for the bulk of care when they fall ill. This can be done either through *insurance* or *exemptions from payments*. Before going on to discuss viable options for pooling within Pakistan, it is useful to know how health insurance and exemption systems are presently configured in Pakistan's health system.

4.3.1 Health insurance

Health insurance can be described under four arrangements in Pakistan's context—social health insurance, private health insurance, community health insurance, and *Takaful*.

Social health insurance: social health insurance refers to a method of covering healthcare costs from funds collected from individuals, employers, or revenues. With the help of these contributions, insurance generally pays a portion of the medical costs of the members secured. Important prerequisites for social health insurance include a mechanism for ensuring compulsory and regular contributions from all of its members and legislation by the government.

Presently, an estimated 6.89 million employees and their dependants are covered under social health insurance arrangements in the country.

Social security, which is one of the five charges imposed by labour legislation on private employers in Pakistan, supports a vertically-integrated insurance scheme under which private employees in a certain low-income category receive healthcare through the health infrastructure of the Employees Social Security Institutes in three provinces—NWFP, Sindh, and Punjab. The institutes use funds generated by employers' contributions to produce services. Many attempts have been made in the past to upscale social health insurance as a means of health financing—details are given in the chapter on the *History of Health Reform* under *Health financing*. However, none of them appeared viable for large-scale application.

Private health insurance: Pakistan has a small private health insurance industry, which has evolved over time. The industry began with service-oriented schemes for major clients by a few insurance agencies in the 1950s. Gathering of data on medical facilities stimulated the development of health insurance schemes for individuals and groups and subsequently group insurance was offered to the corporate sector. The health insurance market is concentrated in the urban areas and owing to its high cost and moral hazard—bogus claims being the main constraining factor—insurance companies have only been able to serve a small market segment.

Community health insurance: most of the community health insurance projects currently underway have been developed by Microfinance Institutions (MFIs). These agencies have used their infrastructure and outreach to underwrite administrative costs and are, therefore, striving to make community health insurance viable for the commercial sector—at least in pilot settings. Most of the currently ongoing projects involve one-time purchase of policies, which MFIs sell to their clients.[250] The National Rural Support Programme (NRSP) and Adamjee Insurance Company's joint scheme targeting NRSP's microcredit clients is an example. None of the projects currently underway has been formally evaluated to date.

Takaful: *Takaful* is a form of insurance relevant to the Islamic society. It is based on the principle of mutual assistance and voluntary contribution and is operated on the basis of shared responsibility. It provides for mutual financial security and assistance to safeguard participants against a defined risk. In conventional insurance, risk is transferred to the insurance company and the surplus is not shared, whereas in Takaful, both risk as well as the surplus is shared—the latter as per the ratio of contribution of the participants. Takaful does not have major share in financing health in Pakistan. Although solutions are currently being offered, there are no data on the number of individuals secured under this scheme.[251]

4.3.2 Exemptions

Pakistan's existing social protection and safety net arrangements—*Zakat* and/or *Bait-ul-Mal*—fund exemptions for poor patients in public hospitals. Theoretically, a local government-certified Zakat certificate entitles the poor to free services where the service involves a user charge in public hospitals. High-cost diagnostic and invasive procedures not funded through Zakat are meant to be financed through Bait-ul-Mal.

Zakat is the Muslim system of charitable contributions to achieve equity in the society.[252] Pakistan has devised a mechanism to institutionally levy Zakat on cash deposits by mandating financial institutions and other collection agencies to deduct Zakat at source and deposit monies in a central fund maintained by the State Bank of Pakistan. From there, funds cascade to the provincial and district Zakat councils and committees respectively, on a population basis. In addition to financing healthcare, Zakat also funds cash transfers to the poor and finances rehabilitation grants and educational stipends. Bait-ul-Mal on the other hand, is an institutional entity set up by the state to help the disadvantaged.[253] It is funded through the federal government budget and provides assistance for a range of programmes. Through its individual financial assistance programme, it underwrites high costs of care—those not covered by Zakat fund—in Zakat-entitled patients.

Despite the existence of elaborate institutional arrangements, Zakat and Bait-ul-Mal contributions account for only 0.45 per cent of the total health expenditure. The relative contribution of both to health, vis-à-vis other sectors, also remains narrow—less than 11 per cent of the total Zakat funds and 8 per cent of the total Bait-ul-Mal funds have been allocated for under-writing healthcare costs over the last 10 years.[254] In addition, the widespread scope for patronage and abuse, discretionary use of power, and exploitation of procedures causes pilferages and mis-targeting, which undermine the effectiveness of these resources. The recently initiated Social Protection Programme of the government of Pakistan is centred on income support and does not include health as an entry point.[255]

4.3.3 Expanding the coverage of pooling

This section of the chapter focuses on exploring options for expanding the base of pooling as a means of health financing in Pakistan, drawing on lessons from around the world.

To date, large-scale government-led national insurance reforms have predominantly been implemented in middle-income countries. Examples include Philippines, Columbia, Chile, and some countries of Eastern Europe. Most of these countries relied on high economic growth rate to expand total health expenditure and levied payroll taxes, which were funnelled into insurance. Examples of government-led insurance reforms in low-income countries include Rwanda and the state of Andhra Pradesh in India. In both these settings, the population base was small and insurance reforms were made possible through injection of significant additional resources. In Rwanda, this became possible with donor support and in Andhra Pradesh, through contributions of the central government of India.[256]

Outside of national insurance reforms, there are examples of experiments in community health insurance mostly by private sector innovators. Examples include pilot models in Ghana, Mali, Senegal, India, Nigeria, Burkina Faso, Bangladesh, and Uganda. In Pakistan, the example of NRSP's pilot project on micro health insurance falls in this category. Countries and international agencies are exploring whether these small-scale efforts have the potential to financially secure poor populations and whether they can be the key point in the evolutionary progress towards comprehensive universal coverage as was the case in OECD countries like Germany decades ago, and as has recently been experienced in Rwanda and Andhra Pradesh.[257]

Pakistan neither has the potential to generate enough revenue in the short-term, nor can it generate the needed level of resources from payroll taxes because majority of its workforce is employed in the informal sector. Hence, it does not appear feasible to advocate for a social health insurance model outside of the formally employed sector.

Recommendations for broadening the base of pooling in Pakistan, therefore, have to be developed in the context of these constraints. This publication suggests a way forward while making a distinction between the formally and informally employed sectors.

4.3.3.i Formally employed sector

For those in the formally employed sector, there appear to be two pragmatic options for broadening the base of pooling. First, it appears feasible for the government to use ESSI as a platform for increasing social health insurance coverage for employees in private commercial and industrial settings and other formally employed sectors; this can be done through statutory changes and modification of qualifying criteria. In tandem, measures need to be undertaken to eliminate abuse and make this vertically-aligned insurance system more effective.

Secondly, an estimated one million individuals and their dependants are covered under private health insurance. The latter plays a limited role in Pakistan as the primary source of coverage because of affordability issues. Growth of private health insurance is correlated with economic growth in general and growth of the formally employed sector in particular. It is only when employers subscribe to global employment practices and factor-in health benefits for a large number of employees that health insurance companies with investment capacities and appropriate domain experience have an incentive to operate in developing countries. By underwriting a large number of people in a pool, they can also create an opportunity, which health providers would wish to avail and may compete for, hence bringing down costs. The government, therefore, needs to analyze the current policy environment for private insurance companies, balancing financial incentives with appropriate safeguards and explore incentives for employers, to encourage them to subscribe. However, in doing so, it should ensure that these measures help to decrease inequities.

4.3.3.ii Informally employed sector

Individuals in the informally employed sector are most vulnerable to health-related shocks. Population-based data from the Planning

Commission of Pakistan show that economic shocks involving catastrophic spending on health are the most common risks faced by poor households in Pakistan. Two-thirds of the households assessed for a safety net survey reported that they had been affected by one or more health shocks and had spent catastrophically during the last three years.[258]

There are two options to pool for financial risk protection to cover the informally employed and their dependants. These include social protection and community health insurance.

Social protection is generally regarded as a mechanism to address poverty and vulnerability by providing protection against uninsured hazards such as illness, unemployment, and disasters, which push vulnerable households into poverty and the poor into persistent poverty. Pakistan's Social Protection Strategy 2005 supports this as a viable tool for illness related financial risk protection, in theory.[259] In reality, however, the existing social protection mechanism—Zakat and Bait-ul-Mal, as already described—has a very narrow base in relation to health. Additionally, it also suffers from governance shortfalls, as a result of which resources get misdirected and pilfered. Therefore, alongside measures to increase the size of the envelope, it is important to mainstream efficiency and transparency in the use of social protection funds.

Creation of a health equity fund is one option to broaden the base of social protection as a means of financing health. An equity pool can be funded through revenues, philanthropic contributions, or donor resources. There are many successful examples of the use of such funds in other developing countries.[260,261] This approach will shortly be pilot-tested in Pakistan through Heartfile's Health Financing pilot project, which will use philanthropic contributions to establish a health equity pool, as described earlier.[262]

Community health insurance is the second health financing option for those in the informally employed sector. Conventionally, the cost implications of administering insurance policies in far-flung rural areas render community health insurance unviable in settings such as Pakistan. However, MFIs in Pakistan are attempting to address this issue by off-setting administrative costs in pilot projects. The example of NRSP's pilot project has already been alluded to. Up-scaling of such a model and building the institutional capacity to administer community health insurance are a daunting task in Pakistan, where institutional ability is limited to cascade pilots into broad-based change. In broadening the base of community health insurance, the potential to leverage Takaful should also be explored.

4.4 Purchasing

When a public or private entity pays a healthcare provider—in the public or private sector—in exchange for curative or preventive services they render to an individual or population, the entity is seen to be 'purchasing' the service as a third party.

The concept of purchasing is inter-linked with the construct of a social welfare and health systems policy. Its introduction into the policy architecture is based on the premise that the role of the state is to finance and ensure provision of services and to provide oversight and that when it comes to the actual provision of services, the system can be organized to harness the capacity of a wide range of organizations and individuals involved in the delivery of care, within and outside of the state system. The approach makes sense in a Mixed Health System, where non-state entities are the major providers of services.

The concept of purchasing becomes clearer when viewed in the context of *vertical* and *horizontal* integration as defined and understood in the world of business science. A health system can also be vertically or horizontally orientated. Simply stated, when agencies both finance as well as provide/produce services themselves, they are said to be 'vertical.' The National Health Service (NHS) type of a health system, the prototype of which is the United Kingdom's NHS, evolved on this pattern. However, over the years, the United Kingdom's Department of Health started purchasing services from private providers—the networks of general practitioners in UK—and therefore became horizontal in terms of service delivery.

Countries such as Pakistan, on the other hand, continue to have a vertical approach to health in the state health system. Other health systems in Pakistan are also vertically-integrated. In the Armed Forces system, revenues are used to produce services while in the Fauji Foundation system, commercial profits are used; the ESSI is an example of a vertically-integrated health insurance system where pooled funds are used to produce services.

Some attempts aimed at strategic purchasing in the health sector have been made in the past. In the late 1990s, the provincial government of Punjab aimed to purchase services from district health authorities under the District Health Government initiative. More recently, district governments have been purchasing services from parastatal agencies—Rural Support Programmes—to manage and provide services in BHUs under the President's/People's Primary Healthcare Initiative.[263] Another example can be cited from the National AIDS Control Programme, which has entered into contractual relationships with NGOs to deliver harm-reduction services to high-risk groups. These examples show that any entity can be involved in purchasing. It is the design of the health system that determines the purchasing agency. For example, in the United States, health management organizations are the major purchasers, whereas in countries where social health insurance is a major means of health financing, a national health insurance organization becomes a major purchaser.

The concept of purchasing is relevant in Pakistan as an option to restructure management of poorly performing FLCFs as has been demonstrated in the contracting out model of PHC, discussed further in the chapter on *Service Delivery*. More importantly, purchasing is also the underlying approach to financing while contracting out the provision of services to existing private health providers. This has been recommended in this publication as one of the options to broaden the base of the state's service delivery arrangements to deliver health-related public goods. Lessons from other countries, where governments have been acting as major purchasers of services from the private sector through competitive contracting, can be instructive in this regard. Examples include the post-conflict countries of Afghanistan, Cambodia, Guatemala, and Rwanda. A similar approach is now being planned for Liberia.[264] However, in these examples, purchasing was straight-forward as there was no entrenched public service. In Pakistan, the case is different as there is an established public service, which despite its weaknesses, consumes a large part of the resources that the government makes available for the health sector and resists any structural change that threatens its interests. Additionally, public employees in Pakistan also have significant protection under the law with respect to their employment status.

Despite these challenges, it must be appreciated that *strategic purchasing* by a knowledgeable organization with appropriate regulatory capacity can offer potential in a Mixed Health System. The challenge would be to create appropriate normative guidance and ensure its implementation through institutional arrangements with the capacity and commitment to make pluralism in service provision work for equity. Here, it must also be recognized that purchasing can be employed as a tool, not only in public-private relationships, but also in government to public sector service delivery agency relationships by employing performance-based financing and incentivizing state actors. These approaches have produced encouraging results internationally, from which useful lessons can be drawn.[265,266]

4.5 Reform of health financing

Reform of health financing within a given setting has to be grounded in local realities. It must take into account, existing sources of health expenditure and pooling, orientation of the health system, the socio-political landscape, and most importantly, the institutional capacity of the country to restructure. Often, radical approaches are recommended for reforming health financing in Pakistan, such as a move towards bringing the entire population under a compulsory insurance scheme. Although the stand-alone merit of this approach is not under question, the institutional and resource prerequisites of such a transformation and the level of dismantling it would entail of the existing system precludes it as a viable option in the short-to-medium term. Such radical measures can be pursued only if Pakistan transforms into a high-resource country with the majority of its workforce in the formally employed sector, a country with stable institutions capable of sustainably implementing major policy change. Until then, reform of health financing will have to centre on a number of locally feasible approaches suited to different settings within the country.

The first priority is to *ensure funding of essential services* by allocating a higher share of revenues for health. Concomitantly, there is the need to *improve returns on spending* by maximizing efficiencies, reducing duplicative costs, minimizing pilferages, mainstreaming innovation, and ensuring that revenue allocation is equitable. Predictable development assistance should be channelled to augment these resources in order to support a consistent and coherent set of nationally agreed objectives in line with stated priorities. Development assistance should be used preferentially to strengthen systems with a view to ultimately transition away from support. In addition, it is critical to promote debt forgiveness as a tool to free up resources for health and other social sectors.

Secondly, there is the need to *pool for financial risk protection* for those in the informally employed sector. Waivers and exemptions funded through social protection funds should be regarded as a critical instrument in this area and measures prioritized to broaden the base of existing mechanisms through the creation of health equity funds. *Appropriate use of technology* can be instrumental in mainstreaming efficiency and transparency in the use of social protection funds. In tandem, evidence from existing pilots of community health insurance should guide up-scaling, where feasible, in collaboration with microfinance initiatives. It is also important to concomitantly build institutional capacity to administer community health insurance.

Thirdly, health financing strategies for those in the formally employed sector should centre on maximizing pooling through insurance. This can be done specifically by using ESSI as a platform for increasing social health insurance coverage for employees in private commercial and industrial settings, and more generically, by making statutory changes and modifying criteria. In addition, there is a need to promote private health insurance, balancing financial incentives with appropriate safeguards, and explore incentives for corporate sector employers in order to encourage them to subscribe. In doing so, it must be ensured that these measures help to decrease inequities.

Lastly, there is the need to *mainstream strategic purchasing* as an option to restructure management of poorly performing FLCFs and as a tool to harness the outreach of private providers. Purchasing should also be promoted in government to public sector service delivery agency relationships by employing performance-based financing and incentivizing state actors.

Chapter 5

Service Delivery

Delivery of health services is one of the key outputs of a health system and ensuring citizens' satisfaction, equity, and quality, one of its goals. A number of attributes of service delivery need to be examined whilst assessing health systems performance. These include service availability, service quality, service utilization, and outreach coverage. The latter two are predominantly relevant to public service delivery.

These attributes are discussed in various sections of this publication. Chapter 2 is relevant to service *availability* as it presents details about the Mixed System of Healthcare, which comprises healthcare infrastructure in the public and market systems. The former includes the Primary Health Care (PHC) infrastructure and public hospitals (Figure 7, chapter 2) whereas the latter includes private ambulatory clinics, dispensaries, and hospitals of various sizes. In addition, a range of individual non-state actors also characterize the Mixed Health System. The description of service availability in this chapter builds further on numeric indicators relating to availability, which the author has described in an earlier publication.[267] The same publication provides quantitative data relevant to outreach *coverage* as well. Data relevant to service *utilization* in the public sector is illustrated in Figure 6 (chapter 2), whilst referring to the predominant relative proportion of care delivered in the market system, drawing on evidence from a cross-sectional nationally representative population-based survey. There are no data presently available to assess service *quality*—a gap which will soon be bridged by evidence from an ongoing assessment of health systems performance, currently being undertaken by Heartfile, as has been described in chapter 2.

This chapter discusses challenges specific to the public healthcare system and malpractices that are common to both the public as well as the market system, and outlines opportunities for reformation of healthcare service delivery in Pakistan.

5.1 Service delivery challenges in the Mixed Health System

Chapter 2 has outlined the determinants of mayhem in the Mixed Health System and Figure 11 in chapter 3 has illustrated the existence of a parallel management system. Figure 13 in this chapter further elaborates upon this through a stylized representation of the manner in which malpractices become institutionalized in public facilities because of structural discrepancies in the Mixed Health System. Low public funding for health and the existence of an active and poorly-regulated private sector and the imbalance, which these factors create in terms of the differences in remuneration and incentives, coupled with lack of transparency in governance, act as a triad in undermining the equity and quality objectives of a health system, as has previously been illustrated in Figure 8 (chapter 2). Low salaries in the public system manifest in the form of a number of individual coping strategies and a range of unethical health provider behaviours. These are exacerbated by absence of regulatory controls and quality assurance mechanisms, poor management, and limited accountability in governance.

Although commonplace, malpractices are by no means solely characteristic of the functioning of the health system in Pakistan. They are rampant in many other developing as well as developed countries around the world. The pattern of malpractices described herein cannot be generalized. Pakistan has many islands of excellence and numerous professionals of high repute and integrity. However, these exist in a system where inefficiencies and malpractices are also widely prevalent and act as major barrier to efforts aimed at improving health status and systems. The nature and pattern of these malpractices need to be understood so that effective and locally suited measures can be structured and sustainably deployed. Of all these malpractices, staff absenteeism, dual job-holding, theft of supplies, and procurement discrepancies are predominantly relevant to public sector healthcare delivery, whereas the broader discussion around unethical behaviours and indifferent attitudes of staff in service delivery and patient care, are common to the public and market system. A brief snapshot of each is provided.

Figure 13. The chain of malpractices in publicly owned health facilities

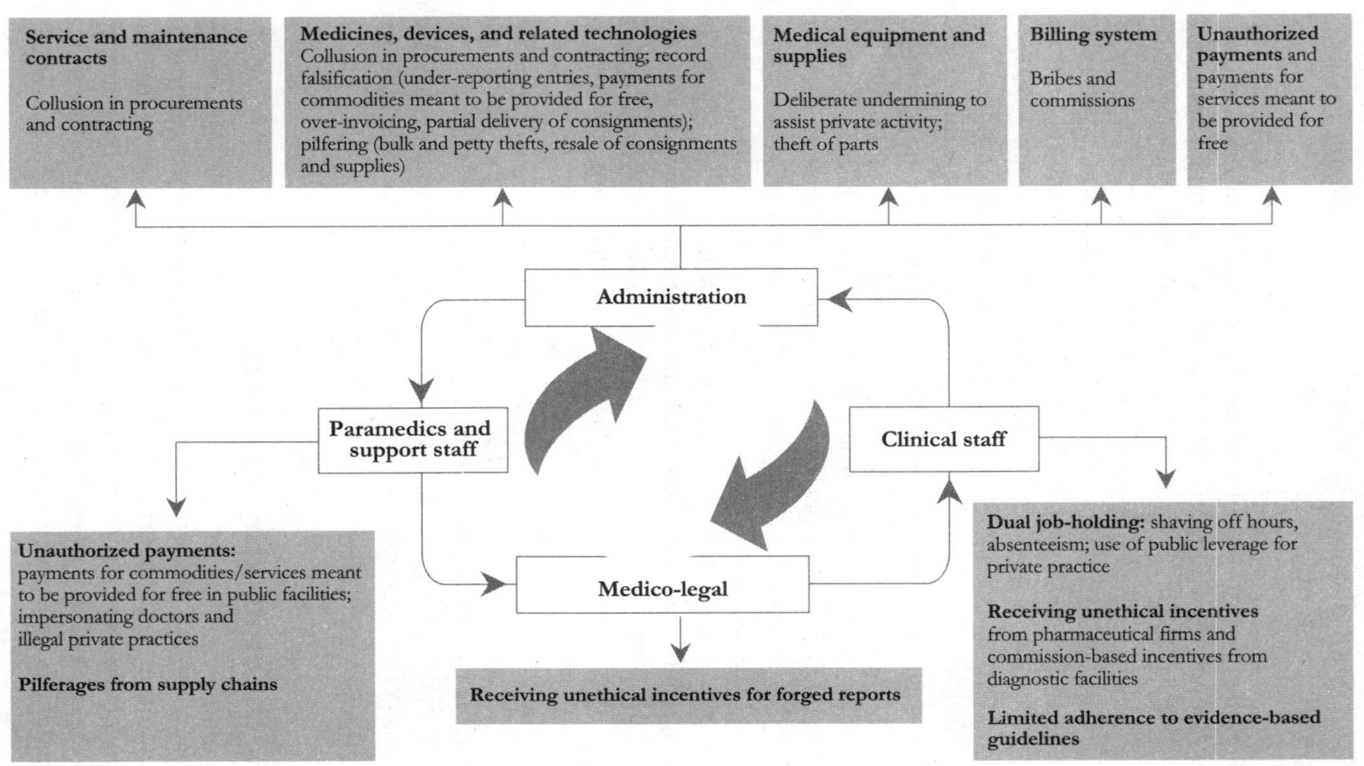

5.1.1 Staff absenteeism and dual job-holding in the public system

Staff absenteeism and dual job-holding by health providers in the public sector and their support staff is one of the commonest issues relevant to public health facilities in Pakistan. Whereas dual job-holding is ubiquitous, staff absenteeism is relatively more common in the case of remotely located First Level Care Facilities (FLCFs), where a certain level of oversight cannot be maintained. In a minority of the cases, absenteeism is unavoidable; for example, rural health workers often need to travel to larger towns to receive their payments, fetch supplies or drugs, and are sometimes delayed by poor infrastructure or weather. However, in most cases, absence is motivated by responsibilities at a second job. Absenteeism and the 'ghost worker phenomenon' are also prevalent in areas where layers of oversight exist, but where institutionalized malpractices create an environment that enables health providers to remain absent from duty in lieu of relinquishing a percentage of their salary, which is shared institutionally. This has been illustrated while describing the Parallel Management System in the chapter on *Governance*. Absenteeism undermines the *equity* objective of publicly financed healthcare as it leads to closed/under-utilized public facilities. It also undermines the quality of healthcare as it often fosters reliance on ill-trained providers in the private sector.

The other staffing issue observed at the higher end of service delivery, particularly in tertiary care hospitals, is hour shaving. This manifests itself as late arrival, early departure, and long breaks. Staff absenteeism and hour shaving can be amenable to service delivery reform where management controls are improved in tandem with strengthening the incentives-performance-accountability nexus.

5.1.2 Unauthorized payments

Unauthorized or informal payment is defined as 'payment to an individual and/or institutional provider—in kind or cash—that is made outside of the official payment channels; these can also involve purchases meant to be covered by the healthcare system. Unauthorized payments include under the table payments to doctors, nurses and/or other medical staff for jumping the queue, receiving better or more care, obtaining drugs, or just simply for any care at all.'[268]

Various patterns of informal payments are known to exist within the public system. As opposed to the commonly described pattern in other developing countries, which usually involves a petty bribe for accessing healthcare, unauthorized payments in Pakistan most commonly involve record tampering and under-reporting of entries. This pattern can largely be attributed to lack of automated systems, as manual records are more readily exploitable.

Absence of automated tracking systems also opens avenues for petty corruption, which enable hospital functionaries to charge costs for medicines and supplies even when these are meant to be provided free of cost. This practice is particularly prevalent in inpatient settings and operation theatres where tracking of supplies delivered by family members becomes difficult. Appropriate use of technology can obviate unauthorized payments of this nature by providing visibility in tracking.

5.1.3 Undesirable healthcare provider behaviours

Pakistan has no dearth of professionally robust and morally incorruptible health professionals. Notwithstanding, malpractices in healthcare provision and healthcare provider behaviours are also rampant, as in any other country. These are being described under two categories.

5.1.3.i Qualified healthcare providers

Doctors employed in the public system are known to unduly use their 'public job leverage' to boost private practices. A number of undesirable behaviours such as reluctance to see patients in public hospitals and 'referral' to private clinics are overtly observed and are almost regarded as a conventional norm. Specialists often collude with their support staff in public hospitals to channel patients to private facilities; support staff is also known to cover up for absences. In most leading public sector hospitals, a specialist's clinic prescription is often the ticket to a hospital bed—a phenomena resident staff is familiar with. These practices continue to prevail despite the existence of a law on private practice and while some of the doctors also draw, what is labelled as the non-practicing allowance on their salary slips.

Quality of care offered in the market system, barring a few notable exceptions, is usually less than desirable due to the tendency to limit investments in inputs. The combination of a number of factors leads not only to compromised quality, but also to blatant violation of patients' rights and medical negligence. These factors include lack of regulatory controls, collusion in oversight, weak tort system, and above all, an environment where consumers of medical services are least assertive about their prerogatives due to illiteracy and general lack of awareness about their rights as patients. No formal studies have been conducted to date to measure quality of care in the private sector. The disconnect between the private sector and the country's Health Management and Information System (HMIS) makes quality enforcement and its monitoring a difficult task, in any case.

No sustained and concerted effort has been made to date, either to regulate the non-state sector or to mainstream its services into the formal channels of service delivery. In the National Health Policy of 2001, one of the 11 areas of focus entailed 'regulation of the private medical sector'. Shortly following this, a draft ordinance relating to regulation of private clinics and diagnostic facilities was circulated to solicit inputs of the civil society.[269] However, it was not subsequently enacted. In the last decade, health regulatory agencies were also created in two out of the four provinces and were mandated with appropriate responsibilities, but have not been able to perform their role. Part of the reason for this relates to the unfulfilled need for a complex set of measures, which need to be set in motion as part of overarching reform of the health system as a prerequisite for creating an environment in which such agencies can function.

5.1.3.ii Non-qualified healthcare providers

Formally trained non-doctors—nurses and paramedics—engage in malpractices by providing services they are not authorized to provide. These and other non-qualified providers—quacks—often impersonate doctors. There are many gaps in regulating such practices and no attempt has been made to date, to mainstream their role into the delivery of care by accrediting them to provide certain services, which on the one hand, can be safe for them to deliver, and on the other hand, can serve as enough of an incentive for them to stay away from delivering services where they are likely to inflict harm. The directions for service delivery reform proposed in this publication call for drawing on the outreach of all categories of healthcare providers. Here, it needs to be explored if quacks currently impersonating as doctors can be made responsible for a certain set of actions within the domain of healthcare delivery. However, concerns relating to the manner in which this will be perceived as an endorsement of their practices, thereby further exacerbating quackery, must receive careful attention.

5.1.4 Pilferage of supplies

The government spends a sizable proportion of its health budget on procuring medicines and related products on the premise that these will be made available to patients free of cost in public facilities. A certain percentage of earmarked resources get pilfered in the process of procurement right at the outset. Once procured and within the supply chain, there are other ways of siphoning off medicines and supplies as a result of a range of administrative malpractices, which include dispensing drugs to ghost patients, padding bills, clever book-keeping, overpayment for supplies, and over-invoicing. Medicines and supplies are also diverted for resale to retailers, wholesalers, or the black market. Instances have been reported where entire consignments have been diverted to the black market for resale. In the Federally Administered Tribal Areas (FATA) of Pakistan, a thriving black market enables peddlers to 'transact' business. The government perceives the use of pre-marked packages 'for government use' a deterrent against these practices. However, staff has been reported to get around this by selling consignments back to the wholesaler.

Other forms of abuse—a result of inefficient management and monitoring capacity—are also well described; e.g., supplies may not meet expected standards, may only be partially delivered, or not delivered at all. It is also possible for low-quality, expired, or counterfeit medicines to be sold in bulk consignments.

In addition to bulk theft, petty theft of medicines and supplies also occurs within the dissemination channel of health facilities and hospitals, largely as a result of the absence of automated systems—manual handling of goods can be more easily exploited. Theft is particularly common in case of items of high commercial value, which are provided free to hospitals. For example, in a radiology department of a tertiary care hospital, a system of pilfering x-ray films is known to exist. Publicly-employed radiology technicians use stolen x-ray films in their 'private practices' and subsequently deposit the films back for proof of use, as the latter is a requirement to ensure that items have actually been used in government-run hospitals.

Equipment spare parts are another high-value item, critically needed for appropriate functioning of sophisticated imaging and diagnostic equipment. Theft of spare parts and their resale in the market is commonplace. In addition, 'the declared malfunctioning of parts' renders public machines out of order, thereby enabling services in the private sector to flourish.

5.1.5 Challenges in prescribing and choosing diagnostic options

Unethical practices in prescribing and choosing diagnostic options for patients are pervasive in the health system. Most of these stem from incentive structures that are either created by marketing practices of the pharmaceutical sector or incentives that the market enables the health provider to generate by subscribing to certain choices in prescribing medicines and choosing diagnostic procedures. This section will briefly address unethical practices in choosing diagnostic options. Malpractices in prescribing medicines and using related technologies have been alluded to in the chapter on *Medicines and Related Products*.

Dual practice of public employees is one of the factors responsible for unethical practices in promoting and choosing diagnostic options. There are anecdotal reports of incidences where managements of public facilities have deliberately impeded certain tests in public hospitals since these are offered at private facilities located across the street.

Some private diagnostic facilities are also known to engage in a range of other malpractices. There is currently no regulation of diagnostic medical equipment and devices in the country. This provides an opportunity to the non-*bona fide* private sector to exploit lack of regulatory oversight by procuring items of low quality—both equipment and disposables—and engaging in diagnostic malpractices in back-office activities. The significant price differentials lead some of them to use low-cost, poor-quality tests while the consumer—unable to decipher the difference—gets charged for a high-quality procedure. In addition, the marketing tactics of diagnostic facilities closely mimic those described for medicines in the respective chapter, where unwritten contracts and pre-arranged kickbacks and commissions with doctors enable laboratories to generate revenue in a highly 'competitive' environment. It is well established anecdotally that laboratories in major cities offer 10–30 per cent in commission to doctors for making regular referrals.

5.1.6 Malpractices in outreach services

A specific pattern of malpractices, which relates to field outreach in service delivery, is endemic to the national public health programmes of the Ministry of Health and the population programme of the Ministry of Population Welfare. These programmes have been slow in impacting outcomes. Immunization rate in Pakistan has stalled at 47 per cent despite the existence of a relatively well-funded national programme, which has been operational for over 15 years now. Similarly, the Contraceptive Prevalence Rate has also stagnated at 29.6 per cent in spite of the existence of a full-fledged Ministry of Population Welfare, geared exclusively to family planning. Owing to the well institutionalized nature of the incentive sharing mechanism, malpractices at the outreach level have prevailed despite efforts by many programme managers and administrative authorities of high repute and integrity to counter them. The population programme's example is being highlighted to show why this has been the case (Figure 14).

The population programme is one of the few adequately resourced programmes in the country, relatively speaking. However, despite that, it has been slow in meeting its objectives. Figure 14 shows that this is partly the result of institutionalized malpractices at the field level, which are geared towards pilfering resources from the system. Collusion between service delivery staff and supervisors fosters deliberate inattention to staff misconduct. As a result, staff remain absent from duty, do not run field operations, and siphon contraceptives for use in private facilities. Service delivery is, therefore, undermined both qualitatively and quantitatively and charges are levied for services that are meant to be provided free of cost. The pattern outlined in Figure 14 is based on anecdotal evidence and cannot be generalized. However, it can be supported by evidence. The recent Demographic Health Survey data on contraceptive mix do not for instance, match service statistics, which emerge from Family Welfare Centres (FWCs).[270]

A similar pattern of malpractices has been observed in the Malaria Control Programme, which employs Communicable Disease Inspectors to carry out the programme's key field activity—spraying of insecticides. Field staff, often party to record tampering, engage in a range of malpractices due to inspectors' deliberate inattention to oversight just as in the case of the previously described example. As a result, insecticides meant for free spraying are sold in the market and the spray equipment put to private use.

Similarly, in the vaccination programme, vaccinators may engage in petty theft in the field at various levels—by charging money for vaccination cards and syringes that are disseminated to them free and/or by selling part of the vaccine stock to private hospitals. The recent Open Vial Policy, where the field vaccinator has the prerogative to open the multi-dose vial even for one child in order to maximize vaccination coverage, is being particularly abused in this connection. Similarly, the TB DOTS programme is abused by forging monitoring visits to draw travel allowances.

5.2 Setting key directions

The previous section has referred to malpractices, which manifest themselves as poorly performing public facilities, low quality services in the public and private sectors, and high out-of-pocket payments for accessing care. Service delivery reform must address these core disparities as a priority. This section outlines additional policy and institutional considerations relevant to service delivery reform within various domains. These focus on revitalizing the state's extensive health infrastructure, leveraging the outreach of non-state actors to deliver

Figure 14. Pattern of malpractices in a publicly financed field outreach programme

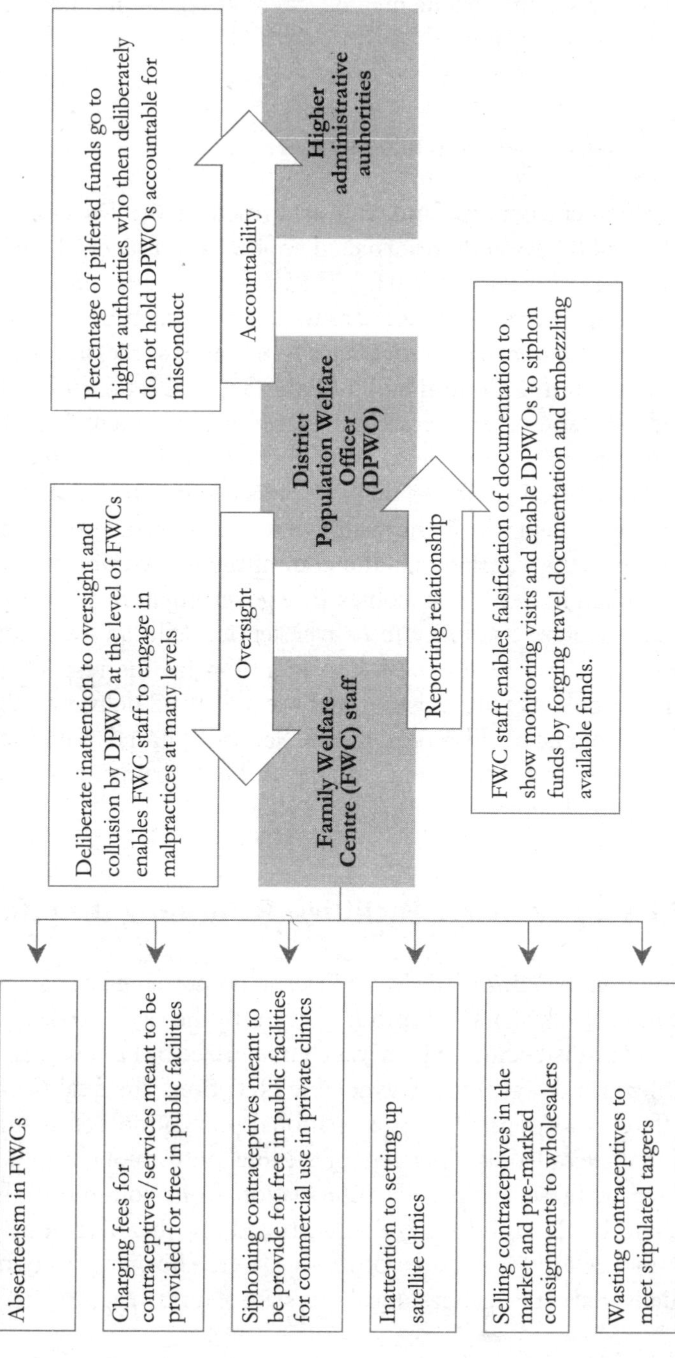

essential services, and introducing non-coercive regulatory measures to foster quality improvement.

5.2.1 Primary Health Care (PHC)

As a development concept and tool enshrined in the Declaration of Alma Ata, and the recently resurrected approach to universal coverage in the World Health Report 2008,[271,272] PHC encompasses both a *set of activities and services to be delivered* as well as considerations relevant to *the first point of contact with individuals.* A review of successive five-year plans of the Planning Commission of Pakistan, health policies of 1990, 1997, and 2001 and other overarching planning instruments—Medium Term Development Framework (MTDF) and the Poverty Reduction Strategy Paper (PRSP)—shows that PHC has featured prominently as a development concept within the health sector in Pakistan over the last 62 years. However, the translation of this commitment into implementation has not resulted in desired outcomes. The government must, therefore, strategically analyze its ability to deliver services and address existing impediments. Three issues merit consideration in this respect. First, addressing problems with existing pathways of PHC delivery—FLCFs and national public health programmes. Secondly, broadening the first point of contact and thirdly, maximizing and optimizing activities and services to be delivered.

5.2.1.i First Level Care Facilities: Reforming the reform

The chapter on the *History of Health Reform* has presented a snapshot of the evolution of Pakistan's PHC infrastructure. By the 1990s, it was evident that the said infrastructure, which was characterized by FLCFs, was being underutilized and that with a few notable exceptions, the quality of care being offered was poor. Data from national population-based surveys showed that overall, only 2 per cent of the total outpatient consultations took place in these facilities.[273] Information from community-based surveys and HMIS additionally demonstrated low turnover of patients per day in FLCFs.[274,275] A range of reasons were shown to account for poorly delivered care—geographical site, state of infrastructure, frequent absence of health providers, paucity of medicines, and lack of referral structures.[276] This realization lent impetus to several attempts aimed at restructuring the management of FLCFs, from the mid-1990s onwards. Notable attempts to restructure management of FLCFs were undertaken under the rubric of the Family Health Project, Social Action Programme, the Sheikhupura project, the District Health Authorities and District Health Government initiatives, and other interventions discussed in the chapter on the *History of Health Reform*.

The recent history of management reengineering of FLCFs is rooted in the Lodhran intervention, an initiative where the department of health of Punjab handed over the management of three BHUs in the district of Lodhran to a parastatal NGO—the National Rural Support Programme (NRSP) in 1999. Based upon the initial encouraging results of this arrangement, the government of Rahim Yar Khan district in Punjab contracted out all of its BHUs to the Punjab Rural Support Programme (PRSP), the provincial arm of NRSP, in 2003.[277] As per the terms of the agreement, the NGO was given the same amount of budget as the district department of health as a single line transfer on a monthly basis. The parastatal NGO was made responsible for management and was given administrative and financial control to implement organizational and management changes. Existing core staff was also made available to the NGO. However, it was not given administrative control over the federally-driven vertical public health programmes. The agreement enabled the NGO to recruit managers on market-based salaries, enhance salaries of medical officers in charge by about 150 per cent, develop community support groups, improve supply of drugs, and upgrade the physical condition of BHUs. The latter was made possible through additional resources made available by the district government. In 2005, longitudinal information from records and a cross-sectional survey in a pretest, post-test, case-control quasi-experimental design showed that contracting had led to increase in utilization at the same overall cost and decreased per-unit cost.[278] However, it had made no impact on improving preventive services, as was expected.

Based on initial results of the Rahim Yar Khan experiment, the approach was expanded to 13 out of the 35 districts of Punjab covering a population of 25 million and was introduced in one-third of all districts of Pakistan as the President's Primary Health Care Initiative (PPHI) in 2003. Weaknesses of the project were not carefully assessed while up-scaling the model. The initiative was hosted by the Ministry of Special Initiatives as opposed to the department of health. As a result, there was lack of ownership of the initiative by the health sector and a counter-productive political turf battle ensued. These problems diverted attention away from the potential within the initiative and the value that partnership with the private sector could bring to management restructuring. In 2008, the new government re-cast PPHI as the People's Primary Health Care Initiative and attached it to the Cabinet Division.

The province of Punjab launched another FLCF management restructuring initiative in parallel with the 'contracting out PRSP model' in 2005 in collaboration with the National Commission for Human Development (NCHD). This model focused on improving services within existing public sector management arrangements.[279] The initiative enabled fresh recruitment of doctors, increase in remuneration and availability of drugs, and upgradation of infrastructure. The programme, which is currently being implemented in 11 districts of Punjab under the Provincial Devolved Social Services Programme, was originally envisaged to strengthen devolution-based management arrangements and has led to some improvements, as is subsequently alluded to. However, as the incumbent government is neither supportive of NCHD nor the devolution initiative—both are viewed as programmes of the previous government—it is not clear as to how this management restructuring arrangement will be sustained, over time.

In summary, as the situation currently stands, 13 out of the 36 districts in Punjab are under an agreement with PRSP. Here, FLCFs are being managed through the contracting out model. In 11 out of the remaining 23 districts, the directly-managed services model is operational in collaboration with NCHD whereas in rest of the 11 districts, FLCFs are being managed, as usual. In the other three provinces of the country, management of FLCFs has been restructured under the contracting out model in less than 30 per cent of all districts. There are, therefore, two restructuring arrangements in place—the contracting out model vis-à-vis the directly-managed services model. A recent study has reviewed both the models through a cross-sectional field survey in Punjab and has outlined both their merits as well as weaknesses and opportunities for further strengthening of these arrangements.[280] In a nutshell, the major strengths of the contracting out model relate to the autonomous status of the managing entity, which translates into quick decision-making, the authority to hire and fire as per need, and flexibility in financial management to create appropriate incentives wherever needed. The programme has two major weaknesses. One relates to its focus on curative care and lack of appropriate integration of preventive services in its scope of deliverables—a weakness the management envisages addressing. The other relates to lack of ownership by the district management, which feels disempowered in this model.

In the NCHD-collaborative reform of directly managed services, on the other hand, there is better district ownership as the EDO Health is the team leader. However, in this case, provincial ownership is weak and managerial and financial flexibilities are limited. The study has shown that in one of the districts evaluated—Gujrat—community participation was stronger than in the contracting out model.[281] The study observed lack of explicit quality of care standards and limited incentives for non-doctor healthcare providers in both the models.

From this analysis, it can be inferred that both the restructuring models have their merits and both can be relevant in different settings. The Ministry of Health and the departments of health in particular have to exercise a stronger stewardship role to translate lessons learnt from these models and develop policy guidance in order to set a direction for management restructuring of FLCFs, which can facilitate the needed upscaling of various models in appropriate settings. The following insights can be relevant in this regard.

First, evidence reveals that lack of capacity and initiative by institutions mandated with health policy-related responsibilities, particularly at the federal level, has been one of the key impediments to initializing reform. This gap has created space for reform to be initialized outside of the official channels of health—the contracting out reform was earlier led by the Ministry of Industries and Special Initiatives and is now housed in the Cabinet Division as opposed to the departments of health. Turf rivalries have additionally posed an impediment to upscale reform. A necessary prerequisite for management restructuring is capacity within health-mandated agencies to initiate and sustain reform, the ability to offer normative guidance and house institutional arrangements at the right level, and the capacity to seek outsourcing management partners through competitive procurement processes. The government must build capacity of its institutions in these areas.

Secondly, the drive to outsource FLCFs should not preclude the option of enhancing efficiency in directly-managed services through managerial reform within the devolved set up by granting comparable levels of financial and administrative autonomy. Purchaser-provider separation and intra-organizational contracting between the department of health as purchaser and the district as provider can introduce elements of competition as an incentive to improve performance and quality. The idea is to strengthen the oversight role of the department of health and to build the capacity of the districts to choose appropriate restructuring arrangements based on locally suited options.

Thirdly, appropriate institutional frameworks should be created to assist with public-private engagement in case of the contracting out model. The chapter section on *Institutional Reform* elaborates on the need to separate policy-making, implementation, and regulatory functions within state agencies mandated in a health role. It makes a case for strengthening the stewardship role of ministries and departments and encourages them to step back from service delivery responsibilities, entrusting the later to autonomous entities, albeit whilst retaining an oversight role. Lessons from the experience of contracting out management in the province of Punjab and existing service delivery arrangements housed under the PRSP can be useful in scaling up and fully housing implementation arrangements in autonomous entities. Ideally, there should be a role for *management* in these arrangements, which can be taken up by the party to which work is contracted out; a role for *quality assurance and evaluation,* which can be taken up by state agencies having appropriate capacity and a role for *community oversight*, which can be served through linkages with the devolution initiative.

Lastly, evidence also underscores the need to match reported levels of efficiency in both the models with outcome results, and therefore, places emphasis on detailing responsibilities compatible with the delivery of a predefined package of essential services as they relate to preventive services and quality of care end-points.

The principles of management restructuring outlined in the *Gateway Health Policy Scaffold*—which has been appended herewith—outline standards with all these considerations in view. Stewardship agencies should enhance their capacities to implement standards and ensure that norms are adhered to, regardless of the mode of management restructuring.

5.2.1.ii Broadening the first point of contact

Existing publicly owned FLCFs have their limitations in serving as the *first point of contact* as envisaged in PHC, given that non-state or private sector actors provide the major bulk of healthcare in Pakistan. This calls for harnessing the outreach of non-state healthcare providers—using relevant management and regulatory tools such as contracting—in order to enable them to deliver essential services. Pakistan has limited experience in involving practicing private sector healthcare providers to deliver health services outside of social marketing and franchising of family planning services.[282] Lessons from these and other successful international experiences should be used to develop a pilot for delivering essential services.

Contracting of private providers can also serve as a market harnessing method of regulating the currently unregulated private healthcare sector in Pakistan. The approach can also enable creation of formal linkages between publicly funded prevention programmes with the private sector, and therefore, enhance the scale and scope of national programmes. This is particularly relevant in case of the malaria and tuberculosis control programmes, which need access to private sector healthcare providers to deliver the clinical components of their prevention and management services.

The broad and inclusive definition of PHC also encompasses the discipline of family practice, which is a relationship-based care that endures over time and over place of care, as opposed to the current public sector PHC model, which is focused on person-to-person care and first-time access. Providers of family medicine can play an important role in delivering PHC, as has been witnessed in Western Europe. Pakistan presently has over 20,000 general practitioners, which remain untapped. With structured postgraduate family medicine training introduced through the College of Physicians and Surgeons of Pakistan, a cadre of family medicine practitioners should be trained and incentivized to effectively contribute to the delivery of essential services over the long term.

5.2.1.iii National public health programmes: Institutional impediments

Salient features of Pakistan's existing national public health programmes and their progress to date, in terms of impact on key outcomes and outputs have been summarized in Table 9. Most of these programmes suffer from a number of challenges, which stem from institutional weaknesses in implementing arrangements and their limited scope. Challenges of healthcare delivery discussed earlier in this chapter also have a deep bearing on the performance of these programmes, since they are implemented through FLCFs. This section will discuss institutional challenges specific to these programmes.

Pakistan's national public health programmes are federally-led with provincial and district implementing arrangements. Other than the National Programme for Family Planning and Primary Health Care, none of the programmes has undergone third party evaluation.[283] Available data from population-based surveys and programme surveillance demonstrate that most of these programmes have had some level of positive impact. However, it is difficult to attribute observed improvements to these programmes because of the inter-dependence of outcomes on a number of factors. The rate of improvements shown varies and has generally been slow. For example, the National Expanded Programme on Immunization, a relatively well-funded programme by local standards, has only been able to increase the percentage of fully-immunized children from 44 per cent in 2002 to 47 per cent, as is presently reported.[284,285] Additionally, issues of capacity appear to be a major impediment. For example, although the LHW programme has had a positive impact on some health outcomes with tripling of LHWs, 30–45 per cent now have low levels of knowledge and skills.[286]

Several factors are responsible for the low rate of improvements. Vertical management, planning, and institutional arrangements of these programmes are an important impediment in this regard. Lack of financial and managerial integration—both across programmes as well as within the district system—has created management anomalies with multiple channels of accountability.[287] Transfer of resources from the federal government to the districts outside of the provincial district accounting and accountability channels has led to lack of ownership of these programmes by the provincial governments. In addition to complicating the management and service delivery system at the district level, these issues are also undermining devolution of power to the district level.

Decentralization of programmes to districts—both administratively and financially—can mitigate some of these challenges. The Ministry of Health should have a normative role in these programmes and should assume responsibility for monitoring and evaluation, technical support, and bulk procurement, the latter only if a cost advantage is gained. Other than these roles, it should empower the provinces and districts to include these programmes in their set of deliverables for health through their regular delivery and accountability channels. This approach can be helpful in addressing the current duplication and fragmentation, to some extent. District integration of programmes can also enable closer control of human resource employed in these programmes.[288] Districts can locally determine and address shortages of technical and administrative staff and frequently reported issues related to training needs and skill development.[289] Decentralization can also mitigate many other programme challenges such as decision-making delays, administrative bottlenecks, and untimely budgetary releases. Devolution of government to the district level in 2001 was envisaged to enable such action. However, devolution has been beset with its own set of challenges as has been described in the section on *Decentralization* in the chapter on *Institutional Reform*. These institutional impediments should be brought to bear in any attempt to restructure the mode of delivering services as part of the national public health programmes.

An important institutional consideration of relevance to these programmes relates to their dependency on efficiently organized FLCFs for effective implementation. Impediments at this level have been elaborated upon in a preceding section of this chapter. Addressing these core disparities is a prerequisite for improving the performance of these programmes. Additionally, any effort aimed at management reform of FLCFs must make a provision for ensuring appropriate linkages with these programmes. The *History of Health Reform* in Pakistan in chapter 2 has highlighted previous attempts aimed at reformation of the PHC infrastructure and has referred to the recent contracting out model, which has shown some level of success in improving efficiency and service update. However, one of the weaknesses of the model relates to the inability of the project's initial design to include preventive services

Table 9. Pakistan's National Public Health Programmes and their impact*

Programme	Description	Impact
National Programme for Family Planning and Primary Health Care Inception: 1994	Delivery of preventive, maternal and child health, and family planning services to women and children by more than 90,000 female community-based Lady Health Workers (LHWs) in the rural areas, covering 55% of the total population of the country.	Independent positive impact on immunization coverage, prenatal care, skilled birth attendants at delivery, and contraceptive prevalence. The third evaluation showed that immunization coverage was 56% and CPR was 30% in LHW covered areas as compared to 38% and 21% in non-LHW covered areas, respectively.[a,b]
Expanded Programme on Immunization Inception: 1984	Provision of immunization coverage against vaccine-preventable diseases to children under one year of age and pregnant women annually; periodic immunization campaigns for other target groups, notably supplementary immunization activities for polio eradication.	Increase in percentage of fully-immunized children aged 12–23 months from 35% in 1990/91 to 47% in 2006/07 and in number of women receiving Tetanus Toxoid during pregnancy from 24% in 1995/96 to 56% in 2006/07.[c] Decrease in the number of polio cases from 1155 in 1997 to 58 as of 2 October 2009; however, transmission of poliovirus still persists and Pakistan is one of the four polio endemic countries of the world.
National AIDS Control Programme Inception: 1988	Delivery of a defined packaged of services to key vulnerable population sub-groups through NGOs; provision of anti-retroviral therapy and screening of blood.	Initiation of service delivery programmes for vulnerable populations and creation of awareness about the epidemic; 78% of the female sex workers know about HIV and AIDS. Change in behaviours, particularly among IDUs and to a lesser extent among sex workers, where service delivery is in place.[d]
National Malaria Control Programme Inception: 1960	Early diagnosis and prompt treatment of malaria; free of cost provision of rapid diagnostic tests at the basic health level, and Artemisinin-based combination therapy for falciparum malaria.	No change in process level indicators over time (Blood Examination Rate and Slide Positivity Rate and outcome level indicators such as Malaria Parasite Incidence Rate and Falciparum Incidence Rate). These data conflict with increasing caseload projections. As a result of data gaps, it is not possible to judge the impact of this programme.
National Tuberculosis Control Programme Inception: 1998	Nationwide implementation of the WHO/IUATLD-recommended DOTS strategy through public sector facilities.	Increase in DOTS coverage from 9% in 2000 to 100% in 2007; Sputum Positive Case Detection Rate from 7% in 2001 to 70 % in 2007, and the Treatment Success Rate from 77 in 2001 to 87% in 2007. Pakistan still lags behind the 70/85 target; high default rate amongst registered TB cases and limitations in including the private sector in the programme pose additional challenges.[e]

Continued...

Table 9. Continued...

National Nutrition Programme Inception: 2002	Implementation of universal salt iodization and fortification of ghee with Vitamin A and wheat with iron and folic acid; enforcement of the Protection of Breast Feeding and Child Nutrition Ordinance.	The number of children stunted, underweight, and wasted has remained relatively stalled at 36.8%, 38%, and 13%, respectively over the last decade; coverage of micronutrients e.g., use of iodized salt, remains low at 17%. Increase in Vitamin A coverage reported.[f]
Prime Minister's Programme for Prevention and Control of Hepatitis Inception: 2006	Mandatory vaccination of all children under one year of age, vaccination of high-risk groups, promotion of safe blood transfusion, disposal of syringes, sterilization of medical devices, and availability of safe water and sewage disposal.	Documentation of hepatitis prevalence through the National Hepatitis Survey—prevalence of Hepatitis B has been reported at 2.5% and that of Hepatitis C at 4.9% in the general population.[g]
National Maternal, Neonatal and Child Health Programme Inception: 2006	Implementation of integrated MNCH services at all levels of healthcare delivery.	The impact of this programme will be assessed over time.
National Programme for Prevention and Control of Blindness Inception: 2005	Strengthening of health infrastructure and up-gradation of technology at secondary and tertiary levels of care; expanding workforce and reinforcing eye care as part of primary healthcare.	Documentation of blindness prevalence through the National Blindness Survey—prevalence of blindness has been documented at 0.9%.

a. Douthwaite M, Ward P. Increasing contraceptives use in rural Pakistan: an evaluation of the LHW Programme. Health Policy and Planning. 2005;20(2):117-23

b. Federal programme implementation unit. Field programme officers' survey 2007: Internal assessment of Lady Health Worker programme. Islamabad, Pakistan: Ministry of Health, Government of Pakistan, 2007

c. Institute of Population Studies and Macro International Inc. Pakistan Demographic and Health Survey, 2006-07. Islamabad, Pakistan: National Institute of Population Studies and Macro International Inc, 2008

d. HIV/AIDS Surveillance Project (HASP), Pakistan. http://jpma.org.pk/ViewArticle/ViewArticle.aspx?ArticleID=1381 (accessed 5 May 2008)

e. National Tuberculosis Control Programme; Ministry of Health, Government of Pakistan, Islamabad, May 2006

f. Bhutta ZA. Maternal and Child Health in Pakistan: Challenges and Opportunities. Islamabad, Pakistan: Oxford University Press; 2004

g. Personal Communication; Executive Director, Pakistan Medical Research Council. Unpublished results of National Survey for Hepatitis Prevalence, 2008

* Some of the programmes are disease specific such as the programmes on HIV and AIDS, malaria, tuberculosis, and hepatitis. Others are specific to the lifecycle domains such as in the case of maternal and child health, whereas others, such as the National Programme for Family Planning and Primary Health Care, National Nutrition Programme, and the Expanded Programme on Immunization are cross-cutting. These programmes present a mixed picture in terms of institutional arrangements and financing, with some being vertical (LHW and nutrition), some already devolved to the provincial level (TB and HIV and AIDS), and others being managed primarily at the districts level (EPI and malaria)

within its realm. Any future effort aimed at improving and upscaling the contracting out model should, therefore, include the deliverables of the national public health programmes in their set of activities that are contracted out.

5.2.1.iv Primary Health Care activities and services

Primary Health Care currently delivers basic curative and preventive services through FLCFs and the national public health programmes. The delivery of services is beset with many challenges as is outlined in the section dedicated to describing the *Challenges in the Mixed System of Healthcare* earlier in this chapter. These impediments need to be addressed as a priority before attention is focused on expanding the scope of activities.

The definition of an optimally suited package of essential health services for Pakistan has to be based on an in-depth technical assessment. In coming to any conclusions, the feasibility of delivery, cost, and acceptability have to be taken into consideration. Past efforts to develop and cost such packages, such as the government of NWFP's initiative to estimate service costs and the more recent initiative of the government of Punjab to develop Minimum Service Delivery Standards, can be used as a starting point to define and cost a package of services.[290]

In developing a package of services, the scope of the national public health programmes should also be reviewed. It must be recognized that these programmes are currently narrow in their scope and have not been attuned to the changing dynamics in public health. Although in recent years, the much needed inclusion of hepatitis and blindness programmes within their remit has broadened their scope, lack of attention to NCDs, injuries, and mental health remains their major weakness—the pilot project initialized for the prevention and control of NCDs in 2003 has not been upscaled. The national programmes also do not address environmental and occupational health. As a result, the negative effects of urbanization, air, noise and chemical pollution, environmental degradation, and agricultural and industrial pollutants, which have a direct impact on the health of individuals and populations, remain outside of the remit of public health in Pakistan. Some of these areas do, however, fall within the ambit of institutional arrangements outside of the health sector. The government should, therefore, be committed to pursuing an MDG+ public health agenda, basing priorities on burden of disease trends as well as the potential for impact within prevention and control efforts. In this connection, due attention should be accorded to emerging health needs in view of epidemiological and demographic shifts.

Developing a package of essential health services also entails synergizing and integrating interventions for diseases with similar risks and common entry points to risk reduction, as the strategy can obviate issues of overlap, duplication of effort, and programme fragmentation. This approach was adopted for the NCD pilot project using common risks—tobacco, diet, and physical activity—as an entry point to address four NCDs in the National Action Plan for the Prevention and Control of Non-Communicable Diseases and Health Promotion in Pakistan.[291] A similar approach can be adopted to integrate HIV and AIDS, and the hepatitis prevention and control programmes, focusing on *risks* rather than *diseases* as entry points. The package of essential services should be able to address a long-standing service delivery disconnect—healthcare and family planning are served by separate institutional hierarchies in Pakistan—by grouping the delivery of family planning services together with comprehensive reproductive health in the essential health services package.[292] Integration of activities will have to be paralleled with integration at the human resource level so that health providers with multidisciplinary skills can be effectively engaged in delivering integrated PHC services.[293] It is, therefore, important to integrate programmes with many perspectives in view.

5.2.2 Hospitals

Several sections of this publication have discussed various aspects related to hospitals, both in the public as well as the private sectors, particularly the former. The description of the *Public and Market Systems* in chapter 1 summarizes details about physical infrastructure. The chapter on the *History of Health Reform* refers to previous efforts aimed at hospital restructuring and reform, as it alludes to key events in the evolution of the health system in Pakistan, whereas the discussion on *Malpractices in the Health Sector* in this chapter is of direct relevance to public hospitals. The section describing the *Parallel Management System* in the chapter on *Governance* additionally describes a pattern of malpractices prevalent in some public hospitals. The pattern has been illustrated further in Figure 13 in this chapter. Similarly, several dimensions of the discussion on human resource and institutional reform outlined in respective chapters, impact the performance of hospitals. This section will discuss past efforts aimed at hospital restructuring and outline key areas for future action.

It is well established that most public hospitals—barring a few notable exceptions—have performance constraints, both in terms of management as well as patient care. Although absence of formal measures to assess the performance of hospitals precludes a precise quantification of inefficiencies, there is anecdotal evidence of major gaps in this area. This realization lent impetus to many initiatives in the past aimed at reforming hospital management. The most notable amongst these was carried out under the rubric of hospital autonomy in Punjab and NWFP. In either case, institutional restructuring arrangements followed the example of successful models of hospital autonomy, globally. Legislation was enacted in either case—the Punjab Medical and Health Institutions Ordinance, 1998 and NWFP Medical and Health Reforms Act 1999. In both cases, Institutional Management Committees (IMCs) were established and Chief Executive Officers (CEOs) were appointed. However, in reality, only a few hospitals benefited from these arrangements and that too, mostly in the area of revenue generation. Institutions in Punjab with smaller administrative units, and those that were able to develop options for institution-based private practice acceptable to all stakeholders, benefited the most. In NWFP, one of the hospitals was able to use its new powers effectively, over time, to generate income and mange its own staff. However, there was no evidence of improvements in quality or equity in access.[294] As opposed to the Punjab and NWFP experiences of hospital restructuring, Sindh focused on emulating the success of one of the institutions, which leveraged innovation and ability to mobilize funds to overhaul management of a specialty hospital.[295]

Limited success of hospital autonomy initiatives in Punjab and NWFP can be attributed to many factors. These stemmed from the restricted financial and administrative autonomy granted under the arrangements and turf rivalries. Even when CEOs were appointed, staff was firmly under control of the department of health, which exercised significant control on staff deployment and undermined—in many cases, inadvertently—efforts on part of the CEO to mainstream accountability. The appointment of CEOs was questioned in many cases on the grounds of merit, capability, and appropriateness. In any case, performance agreements were not clearly stipulated. Additionally, there was lack of clarity—particularly in NWFP—in terms of the functional boundaries between hospital Medical Superintendents, who continued to exercise control, and the CEOs.

Financial arrangements were another impediment. Although hospitals that were made autonomous were given a one-line budget and the flexibility and leeway to reappropriate budgets, they were not allowed to retain 100 per cent of the revenue. This was a major barrier to performance as the administration and staff had no incentive to enhance efficiency. In many cases, the health department was still empowered to order financial, medical, and managerial monitoring. This was sometimes used as a coercive tool and proved to be counter-productive. Hospital information system constraints, except in a few individual units, were also a barrier to ascertaining progress and pitfalls. Improvements in process indicators, as were claimed, could therefore not be ascertained and documented. In addition, because of limited management capabilities, many hospitals were unable to develop comprehensive sustainable business plans. As a result of all these factors, most of the hospitals were not able to successfully mainstream a corporate culture, as was envisaged. Introduction of user's fee was a further complicating factor, which in the absence of comprehensive parallel exemption systems, created a negative perception about hospital autonomy. As a result of all these drawbacks, there has been a lack of motivation to take the hospital autonomy initiative forward, particularly in NWFP, where it has attained a negative connotation. Additionally, status quo is also in the interest of some stakeholders.

Any new attempt aimed at hospital reform must now begin with a careful analysis of existing evidence. The impediments to earlier reform initiatives must be addressed in order for reform to be successful in the first place. Questions to be addressed in this regard fall outside of the purview of the health sector and hence complicate the situation. How can hospitals be empowered to retain revenue when the Auditor General of Pakistan's rules prohibit state agencies from doing so? How can employees, who are recruited for a 35-year contract with limited accountability with reference to performance, be made accountable to hospital CEOs who are themselves contractually employed? How will it be ensured that hospital management is truly capable of mainstreaming private sector entrepreneurial talent, but will at the same time be sensitive to considerations of equity? How will merit-based recruitments come about to ensure that managers with appropriate competencies are in place and how will we guard against crony appointments in such lucrative positions in today's environment of governance? Where is the money to hire such human resource in view of the current financial constraints facing Pakistan in the first place? How will the departments of health and the Ministry of Health distance themselves from micromanaging and divest human resource and financial management controls, given the pervasive culture of patronage? What is the capacity of these agencies to exercise oversight and ensure that corporatized hospitals do not just pursue incentive-driven efficiency as a goal-post, but also serve the needs of the poor? How will we cast hospital reform in the context of reform of health financing to ensure that the right exemption systems are in place so as to offset the risk to the poor in accessing care in hospitals that levy a user fee? All these questions need to be addressed before we can renew and recast a plan for reformation of public hospitals.

In this entire discussion about hospital reform and autonomy, it is important to remember that the ultimate outcome of this effort is to promote quality of care and equity in access—making hospitals autonomous; the focus on efficiencies and private sector management skills is, therefore, just a means to an end.

5.2.3 Behaviour change communication

Individual behaviours with reference to health and healthcare are dependant on a number of factors. These include cultural, religious, social and individual values, beliefs, perceptions, and attitudes. Individual lifestyle, treatment-seeking and compliance behaviours as well as health provider behaviours have an important bearing on the performance of a health system and should be leveraged to bring about improvements within the system. A number of approaches can be used to influence behaviours. These fall on a spectrum and can range from non-coercive to coercive approaches and include communication, incentives, information dissemination, marketing, restriction, indoctrination, and prohibition. Behaviour Change Communication (BCC) traditionally deals with the communication and information dissemination aspects of behaviour change.

The Ministry of Health and the departments of health allocate significant resources to support BCC campaigns through the media. It is, therefore, important to maximize their impact by broadening the scope of health communication beyond the public service announcement approach. This can be achieved by drawing lessons from behavioural research in areas such as persuasion and large group processes. Additionally, social marketing can be used as a tool to complement health reform initiatives. Behaviour change communication should be systematically oriented around a number of social, cultural, and individual perceptions and beliefs that determine health-related knowledge and behaviour, capitalizing Pakistan's tightly knit community structure. There is also a need to target all categories of individual behaviours and to synergize BCC interventions in the health sector with other related interventions—such as family planning—in order to impact the behaviour of all actors in the health system.

5.2.4 Payment mechanisms

Financial incentives are amongst the most important influences over organizational and individual behaviour in a health system.[296] However, payment mechanisms and the means of using them as incentives have to be taken into consideration in the context of how a health system is organized. For example, in Pakistan's revenue funded public system, there are two levels of payment. At the first level, payments are made from the federal government to the provinces and districts; these are usually made on historical grounds, based on traditionally used criteria such hospital-bed ratio. At the next level, when payments are made to staff, they are usually in the form of salaries. A fundamental shift in these payment mechanisms from the traditional historical criteria to hospital performance-based criteria and from salaries to salary plus bonuses can incentivize performance enhancement.

Setting the right payment systems is a sensitive affair and there are pros and cons of any option. For example, if payments to public providers are too low, providers will opt out of government-financed systems, charge additional amounts to patients, or seek under the table payments, as is currently being observed in Pakistan's Mixed Health System. Conversely, if payment levels are too high, the results can be unacceptable. In insurance systems, fee for service can lead to over-services and payment by capitation can lead to under-servicing. The choice of payment in any health system setting, therefore, has to be based on a careful analysis of market and regulatory factors and the envisaged resulting distortion, which can be most amenable to oversight.

5.2.5 Innovations in service delivery

In recent years, there has been a growing realization of the potential within marketing products and services to those at the bottom of the pyramid—the poor who live on less than US $1–2 a day.[297] The mobile phone industry has been particularly successful in this regard through the creation of low-margin, high-volume rugged versions of products suitable for harsh settings. Through this approach, they have been able to capture a wide market segment and have put mobile phones in the hands of a large number of people, even in countries such as Pakistan where more than a quarter of the population lives below the poverty line, but where 58 per cent own mobile phones. Successful examples of double bottom line institutions, particularly microcredit enterprises, have also developed services for the poor on the premise that they are bankable. This approach has led to the burgeoning of a successful industry with a social mission and an unprecedented increase in the number of people who now have access to credit and an opportunity to improve their standard of living.

The social sector in general and health in particular need to learn from these examples. Within the health sector, there are only a handful of service and product delivery innovations that cater to the poor.[298,299] The most illustrative example of this is the case of Aurolab, which now sells an intraocular lens for US $5, supplying 10 per cent of the world's demand. Other innovative financing strategies, delivery processes, and experiences with franchising are also being used as strategies for scale-up.[300,301] The development of viable low-cost innovations in services delivery and product development, if coupled with appropriate government subsidies and facilitation and/or support for upscaling, can be a critical tool in improving affordability, availability, and costs to the poor. The potential to mainstream these into social sector systems needs to be carefully explored in Pakistan's environment.

5.3 Trade in health

Before a synthesis of the directions of service delivery reform is summarized in the concluding section of this chapter, the trade-health nexus merits special attention with reference to service delivery and the need to synchronize the two within that remit. Some dimensions of this discussion are also relevant to human resource regulation.

The World Trade Organization's General Agreement on Trade and Services and a majority of the regional trade agreements allow countries to undertake commitments in trade and investments in health services, if they so desire and in line with their own policy objectives. However, in the Uruguay Round and in subsequent session negotiations, the lowest number of commitments by WTO members was in the health sector and not a single health-negotiating proposal was advanced in the Doha development agenda.[302] Despite this, cross-border trade in health in countries such as Pakistan is burgeoning under the combined influence of a number of factors. Four modes of trade in health need to be taken into consideration while developing and synergizing health and trade policies.

First is the area of cross-border supply of health services. This is a result of the twentieth century information communication technology boom, which has created opportunities for business process outsourcing. Within the domain of health, Pakistan has become an option for low-value offshore back office healthcare services such as medical transcription and billing owing to low cost of labour. High-value remote diagnostic and reporting services are limited due to the absence of regulatory frameworks and inadequate international marketing capacity of Pakistani companies—a gap, which Pakistan's trade policy must address. Overall, the 'outsource' industry has had a positive impact on employment generation. However, it has not added value to healthcare in the country in terms of fostering improvements in quality through the spill-over effect, as has been observed in many other countries. The potential within that must be explored.

The second mode of trade in health is consumption of healthcare services overseas. Many Far Eastern countries have leveraged the potential therein to improve their health systems, which then become an important source of foreign exchange and add to the multiplier effect of tourism-related activities in the economy. This type of trade in services has taken an undesirable route in Pakistan, as in many other developing countries, with burgeoning of kidney transplant tourism.[303] In 2007, the Transplantation of Human Organs and Tissue Ordinance, 2007 was promulgated.[304] The ordinance has lapsed as it was not ratified by the National Assembly nor was its term extended. The ordinance suffered from many weaknesses as it stood. Recently, a revised version of the bill has been tabled. This version has further weakened certain covenants of the law.

It must also be recognized that medical tourism has limited potential in Pakistan for a number of reasons. The success of medical tourism depends on many factors. These include high degree of sophistication of indigenous health systems, high quality of healthcare at relatively low cost, an expatriate friendly environment, and a well developed tourism industry. Based on these criteria, it is clear that the medical tourism industry would not have an emerging trend in Pakistan at least in the short to medium term. It is, therefore, important that public resources earmarked for health should not be used to promote medical tourism at the cost of services that are more equitable.

The third mode of trade in health involves the commercial presence of a foreign service provider in a host country for the purpose of supplying health services. Pakistan is the sixth most populous country in the world and a large market. If the country's overarching environment is conducive, investments in the healthcare sector from off-shore sources are likely to increase, particularly since governments have traditionally been promoting policies favouring liberalization of services in the public domain. While this approach is beneficial in terms of upgrading healthcare infrastructure, generating employment, and providing specialized services, it can also lead to inequalities by creating a two-tiered health system with high-quality care being supplied to the affluent. Trade and health policies should, therefore, balance incentives for investments with appropriate safeguards.

The fourth mode of trade in health services relates to migration/ movement of health professionals out of the country. Such movements can exacerbate existing health workforce shortages, as is currently being observed in the case of nurses, paramedics, and public health professionals in Pakistan. The current doctor-nurse ratio has been 2.7:1 for some time as opposed to the recommended 1:4. Despite this, more than 1800 nurses trained at state expense have moved out of the country over the last five years.[305] The priority should be to meet health workforce needs of the country through appropriate retention arrangements as opposed to a focus on export on the premise that the latter generates foreign remittances.

The WTO Agreement on Trade Related Intellectual Property Rights (TRIPS) is another consideration of relevance to the trade-health interface. This aspect of trade in health has been discussed in detail in the chapter on *Medicines and Related Products* under *Intellectual Property Rights Regulation*. The interest in this area in Pakistan stems largely from the focus on export of generic drugs with which trade in health is closely identified. However, it must be recognized that there are other more important considerations with respect to the TRIPS-health interface—in particular, making use of flexibilities granted under the Doha Declaration on Public Health, where attention needs to focus.

In view of all these considerations, it is important to see trade in a holistic manner and broaden its scope from commodities to the entire value chain, including services and human resource. Appropriate covenants in health and trade policies need to be developed and synchronized to ensure that trade norms maximize equitable health benefits and minimize risks, especially for poor and vulnerable populations. Because of its specificities, health services and human resource should feature as separate items in Pakistan's national trade policy.

5.4 Service delivery reform

Although the private sector plays a predominant role in delivering health services in Pakistan, it must be recognized that the state has both the mandate as well as the responsibility to ensure provision of essential services on a universal basis, with equity as a core consideration. It is important that the state does not divest from this responsibility while reforming the mode of service delivery. Within this context, there are a number of imperatives for service delivery reform.

The first priority is to address current malpractices in service delivery at all levels. Reform of instruments of governance and structural processes of the state discussed in the respective chapters assume great importance in this regard. Without attention to these, isolated service delivery restructuring will have limited impact.

Secondly, there is the need to expand the focus of Primary Health Care, both with reference to the *set of services to be delivered* as well as *the first point of contact with individuals.* In terms of the former, a set of MDG+ essential services should be benchmarked as a yardstick for public delivery and as the basis of contractual relationships with non-state actors. In addition, the national public health programmes should be integrated with the provincial district accounting and accountability channels. In order to expand the first point of contact and augment coverage, restructuring of PHC should centre on contracting existing non-state providers in the short term and training a cadre of family practitioners, over the medium-to-long term.

Thirdly, it is important to restructure the management of state-owned public facilities in order to enhance their performance. The policy on restructuring must take into account, evidence from existing initiatives and ensure that the restructured system has checks and balances with designated roles for management, quality assurance and evaluation, and community oversight. The policy should additionally strengthen decentralization and allow for evidence-based locally suited options to be adopted.

In the fourth place, there is the need to ensure that any attempt aimed at reforming hospitals is centred on improvements in quality and equity. In order to meet these objectives, governance and management in hospitals should be truly decentralized, albeit with appropriate safeguards and inclusion. User fee, where absolutely necessary, should only be used as an incentive for quality but not at the cost of creating access issues for the poor. In such settings, public resources should be used to support objectives that directly serve the equity objective.

In the fifth place, several other factors, which can support reform of FLCFs and hospitals, should be given due consideration. These include strategic use of BCC, social marketing and payment mechanisms. Innovations need to be additionally explored in service delivery in order to reach the hardest-to-reach segments of the population. In addition, market harnessing methods of regulation that foster peer oversight and accreditation, using quality as a benchmark, should gradually replace the command and control style of regulation.

Lastly, Pakistan's trade policy should articulate trade norms in order to maximize equitable health benefits and minimize risks, especially for poor and vulnerable populations. Because of its specificities, health services and human resource should feature as separate items in Pakistan's national trade policy.

Service delivery reform, as envisaged in these directions, needs to be dovetailed and synchronized with reform of financing. These changes necessitate astute institutional capacity for implementation and a sustainable long-term vision in order to be successful.

Chapter 6

Health Related Human Resource

Human resource and health systems are deeply interwoven. Human resource is not just another input into the health system, as are financial and physical resources. Individuals are strategic actors within the system who can act individually or collectively to facilitate the process of reform by improving quality and efficiency. Conversely, they can also be the critical impediment to a reform process.

Reform in most health systems domains is closely interlinked with human resource performance and vice-versa. For example, decentralization can grant appropriate prerogatives and/or take away decision-making powers that promote arbitrariness.[306] Outsourcing can impact working conditions and new service delivery arrangements can either be perceived as a threat or present a conducive environment for enhancing performance. Public-private redeployment and new recruitment and retention mechanisms, and empowerment of facilities by granting autonomy can have implications for incentives and, therefore, impact staff morale and performance, whereas changing public service status can spark strikes and demonstrations as it can have implications for workload and incentives. Implementation of NWFP's hospital autonomy policy in 2002 is a case in point as it led to widespread protests by paramedics, who feared losing their flexible public job status by being part of a more stringently governed private sector.[307] Reform in many health systems domains can, therefore, impact performance of human resource. On the other hand, changes in human resource policies can also assist with or be an impediment to the reform process.

This chapter should be read in conjunction with three other sections. First, the section on the *Public management process* and the *Parallel management system* in the chapter on *Governance*. These discuss the role of the public sector in the set of processes that deal with human resource, in particular anomalies of decision-making in recruitments and placements and issues prevailing at the oversight and accountability levels. Secondly, the section on *Service delivery challenges* articulated in the previous chapter, and thirdly, the section on *Regulation of health-related human resource,* also discussed in the chapter on *Governance.* These have a major bearing on human resource management in the public and private sectors. This chapter will address aspects of human resource management relevant to service delivery workforce and health administration.

6.1 Service delivery workforce

This section discusses three issues in relation to service delivery workforce—numerical inadequacies, issues related to distribution and deployment, and problems with capacity building and training.

6.1.1 Shortage of health related human resource

Healthcare provider-population ratio assessments that benchmark international recommendations and comparative assessments of corresponding workforce-population ratios in neighbouring countries provide evidence of numerical inadequacies in many categories of health-related human resource in Pakistan. It is well-established that numerical inadequacies are particularly pronounced in the case of dentists, midwives, nurses, laboratory, surgical and anaesthesia technologists and assistants, pharmacists, biostatisticians, appropriately qualified health management specialists, and environmental and public health experts.[308]

Numerically, the situation is relatively better in the country as far as doctors are concerned. This can be ascribed to decades of focus on producing more doctors in successive five-year plans of the Planning Commission of Pakistan. Even though the current doctor-population ratio of 1:1326 is lower than the WHO-recommended ratio of 1:1000, increase in the number of doctors from a few hundreds in 1947 to 121,374, as is presently reported, represents an ascendant trend and is favourable compared to many other developing countries. However, the implications of providing more doctors for the healthcare system are seldom analyzed and the establishment, number, and location of medical schools and their seats, in particular, are usually determined, not by the needs of health services but largely by political expediency. In comparison, other areas such as capacity building, training, and effective deployment of doctors have received little attention over the years.[309]

A number of factors are responsible for numerical inadequacies. First, shortages related to dentists, nurses, midwives, pharmacists, laboratory technicians and environmental, public health, and health management experts in Pakistan are mainly due to lack of investment and attention and inability to regard these areas as a priority in health systems management and overall policy level decision-making over the last several decades. Human resource targets stipulated in various strategic planning documents are rarely based on assessment of healthcare provider ratios, nor are any subsequent measures taken to allocate resources on a sustained basis to augment workforce in critically-needed areas. For example, the current doctor-nurse ratio has been 2.7:1 for some time—evidence, which should have guided concerted action to bridge this wide gap in view of the recommended doctor-to-nurse ratio of 1:4. Recently, measures have been taken to increase the number of nurses by incentivizing the private sector to train nurses and underwriting costs of training in private nursing schools. Such strategies must be paralleled with regulatory measures to retain workforce in the country, if the objective is to augment numbers. Similarly, it is well known that all the training institutes put together can provide less than 2000 pharmacists per year—a capacity in stark contrast to need. There are over 50,000 pharmacies in the country with less than 2000 employing qualified pharmacists.[*] A concerted effort has long been overdue to enhance training capacity and improve retention policies. Appropriate action has not been forthcoming in both areas.

Secondly, the issue of inadequate numbers in the public sector is compounded by high attrition rate and migration both to urban centres, private sector, official development agencies, and NGOs within the country as well abroad where better incentives are offered. In recent years, the issue of migration has also been exacerbated by movement as a result of the poor law and order situation. These factors notwithstanding, lack of appropriate remuneration and adequate incentives for performance remain the key factors responsible for numerical inadequacies.

Thirdly, shortages in a particular setting are often purely linked to administrative constraints imposed by inadequate sanctioning of posts or inability to fill a vacant post. The government can begin to address this issue by analyzing local administrative constraints in various settings. Lastly, it is often stated that aggregate numbers also suffer due to women enrolling but not subsequently pursuing careers. Whilst there is anecdotal evidence of this trend, its true impact on numbers remains to be determined. Better opportunities for women and conducive working conditions can help address this barrier.

Numerical inadequacies are usually not easily traceable because of lack of consolidated human resource databases in the country. None of the health information systems currently operational in Pakistan collects information on human resource numbers. Available information comes from accrediting and regulating agencies such as the Pakistan Medical and Dental Council, Pakistan Nursing Council, Pakistan Pharmacists Council, etc. However, since registration in these institutions is at the discretion of health professionals, databases are usually incomplete as many, especially those who serve in the private sector and others not pursuing academic interests, do not appreciate the need to register themselves. All the above-mentioned factors interplay to compound human resource shortages.

6.1.2 Mal-distribution and ineffective deployment

Producing more healthcare providers and investments in training and capacity building can only impact health outcomes if the workforce is effectively deployed, given adequate incentives, and managed efficiently. Previously described numerical inadequacies are compounded by mal-distribution, ineffective deployment, and uneven distribution between the rural and urban areas. Therefore, alongside measures to address quantitative and qualitative discrepancies, attention should focus on effective deployment of human resource.

A number of factors are responsible for mal-distribution of human resource. Foremost is the lack of incentives, which prompts providers as well as health administrators to serve in the private sector or seek employment overseas, where better incentives are offered. Many amongst these continue to hold public sector jobs, even in absentia. In addition, other determinants of low numbers discussed previously also play a part in accentuating workforce mal-distribution.

Poor infrastructure of public health facilities—most notably FLCFs—contributes to mal-distribution as it drives providers away from rural and peri-urban areas to larger towns and bigger facilities. It has been shown that a large number of FLCFs do not have basic amenities—water, electricity, and public toilets—and are not accessible through roads.[310] In addition, irregular supply of medicines and other provisions, weak team management, absence of financial authority, inefficient referral support, and unsafe working environments are also an impediment. These factors are compounded by lack of non-financial incentives such as opportunities to train.

The government needs to take a number of steps in order to overcome numerical shortages and workforce mal-distribution. As a starting point, it needs to develop a comprehensive human resource policy based on an objective assessment of needs. Secondly, the feasibility of enacting a Health Services Law should be explored. Legislation can encompass all categories of healthcare providers. It can define career structures and job descriptions, outline reporting relationships and tenure policy as well as lay down service, promotion, and recruitment rules. The law can also review cadres with a view to eliminating duplication and overlap, as for example, in the case of Lady Health Visitors, Midwives and Family Health Workers. In this case, a cadre of workers with multidisciplinary skills can address shortages as well as obviate issues with disease specific health workers. Review of cadres in other areas can similarly prove helpful. The most important objective of any health service-related legislation should be to help inculcate a culture of merit, performance, and accountability.

6.1.3 Training and capacity building

Education, training, and capacity building should be the centrepiece of Pakistan's human resource policy. Many issues need to be addressed in the domain of undergraduate and postgraduate education, in-service training, and continuing education. Each of these has to be relevant to the needs of respective health professionals.

A few issues warrant urgent attention. Foremost is undergraduate education, the curriculum and format of which needs revision in view of contemporaneous needs and locally suited priorities. Although a few medical schools are currently experimenting with innovative teaching approaches, these have not been widely institutionalized. Postgraduate education, though comparatively better organized, focuses exclusively on specialty care. There is almost no emphasis on developing and incentivising a cadre of practitioners of family medicine who can play a role in assisting the state in delivering services as is described in the chapter on *Service Delivery*. Furthermore, there is no structured system of Continuing Medical Education (CME), particularly for doctors. This huge gap is bridged by the pharmaceutical sector where CME in the name of sponsorships for conferences raises many conflict of interest-related concerns. In the case of nonphysician healthcare providers, institutional mechanisms for CME and in-service training exist in the form of District Health Development Centres. However, these are being used increasingly by NGOs for *ad hoc* trainings, in specific themes, as a result of which healthcare provider training is moving away from the concept of integrated PHC. In view of some of these gaps, the government should explore possible priorities for reforming education, training, and capacity building. The following measures can be important in this regard.

Firstly, as a starting point, a policy should be formulated to guide reform of undergraduate and postgraduate education, training, and continuing education after an appraisal of factors that determine quality of medical education and the impact of privatization on quality. The policy should address faculty issues and governance and administration of institutions, and pay due attention to their de-politicization and establishment of accreditation systems. Secondly, there is the need to update undergraduate medical education curricula both in terms of content as well as in terms of the mode of teaching. In terms of content, primary, preventive and promotive community and public health perspectives need due attention. In addition, there is also a need to broaden the scope of curricula to cover subjects such as health systems management, social mobilization, and the inter-sectoral scope of health. In terms of format, the focus needs to shift towards problem-based learning and competency based education. Priority training needs of postgraduate education should be determined in partnership with the Higher Education Commission. Furthermore, in-service training of all categories of healthcare providers should be strengthened by institutionalizing professional self development. The feasibility of making specified credit hours of CME training a mandatory requirement for promotions as well as a criteria for renewal of registration by appropriate professional bodies should also be explored.

6.2 Human resource dimension of health administration

Human resource is critical to health administration and underpins the viability of any institutional reform. However, as opposed to this and as discussed in the chapter on *Governance*, human resource issues are widely prevalent in the public management process.

This section will discuss health related human resource issues under three areas—staffing key governance positions, training and capacity building and institutionalizing accountability.

6.2.1 Staffing key governance positions

There are three issues in staffing key governance positions in the health sector. First is the issue of capacity, as has been discussed in a subsequent section of this chapter. Secondly, inability to offer market-based incentives is often cited as an impediment to recruiting and/or retaining appropriately trained and qualified health systems administrators and public health specialists within the public sector. Inflexibility of public rules is always regarded as a key bottleneck in this regard. However, there are examples of public sector institutions that have overcome these constraints while remaining within the confines of public sector regulations. For example, the National HIV and AIDS Control Programme has been offering market-based incentives to staff and consultants from Public Sector Development Programme resources. Other public sector institutes that have been granted autonomy through acts of Parliament have also been able to incentivize salary structures, as in the case of the Health Services Academy. In the case of academic institutions, the Higher Education Commission's Tenure Track

Policy should be able to support incentive-building programmes.[311] Flexibilities and appropriate provisions within the public system should be capitalized to institutionalize appropriate incentives, as these are an important motivational factor in staffing key governance positions.

Thirdly, most of the health administrators and senior managers in technical administrative roles in the Ministry of Health and the departments of health do not belong to the civil services cadre. For this category of staff, there are no career paths. Additionally, there are issues related to tenure security and incentives. These factors act as an impediment to retaining human resource within the state's administrative system. In 2007, recommendations of the National Commission for Government Reform (NCGR) developed options to address this gap. The commission was created in 2002 as a high-level statutory body and was tasked with the responsibility of developing recommendations to reform the executive branch of the state.[312] After a series of deliberations, the commission reached a consensus over the broad principles underlying institutional reform. These principles fall under three domains—civil services structure, structures of the federal, provincial and district governments, and business process re-engineering.

The commission's recommendations called for the establishment of a National Executive Service (NES) with the objective of creating streams of professional civil servants to staff policy formulation and key governance positions at the federal level. The structure was meant to cascade from the federal to the provincial levels, over time. Social sector management was classed as one of its four categories. The NES was meant to facilitate appropriate deployment in key governance roles. In concert with other NCGR recommendations on selection processes, career paths, tenure security, training, and compensation, the NES was meant to incentivize public service. Other NCGR recommendations to streamline and optimize rules of business were meant to enhance efficiencies. Recommendations of the NCGR have not been implemented to date and appear to have been shelved.

6.2.2 Training and capacity building

Training and capacity building should be a lifelong process for personnel in administrative ranks. It should ideally be conducted in an environment of policy research at pre-service, induction, refresher, mid-career, and senior levels in common and specialized areas and in technical and soft domains.

Issues of capacity predominantly stem from lack of appropriate training. The colonial-contemporary lag—described in the chapter on *Governance*—also accounts for the capacity gap. Majority of the officers serving in the federal and provincial governments, who do not belong to any cadre or service, are not systematically trained; their technical and managerial skills, are therefore, not upgraded. This has a negative impact on the quality of governance. Plans were previously made to institutionally reorganize training and capacity building for ex-cadre officers at the federal and provincial levels. However, these have not been implemented.[313]

For civil servants who belong to established cadres, a sustainable avenue for capacity building can involve the incorporation of appropriate guidance into the curricula of schools of public policy. On the other hand, short courses that are inspirational, transformational, and catalytic in nature can also be instrumental in enabling career shifts and interests towards health systems. Similarly, capacity building and knowledge enhancing modules can be developed for those in leadership and policy-making roles. These should be offered, not just to ministers who have a rapid turnover, but also to parliamentary committees and political parties in order to maximize the institutionally sustainable effect on building capacities and competencies.

6.2.3 Institutionalizing accountability

The third and most important issue in the public management process concerns the interrelated attributes of poor performance, inefficiencies, collusion, and lack of transparency in decision-making. These can be attributed to poor structures of accountability, the pervasive culture of patronage, and political interference. The chapters on *Structural Reform of the State and Health* and *Governance* outline specific measures, which can help institutionalize transparency and promote efficiency within the state system in general and the health system in particular. Within this broader remit, the need to institutionalize integrity in public service is of particular relevance to reform of health administration. Although integrity is envisaged to be an attitude, there are means of structurally inculcating it such as by developing systems of compensation adequate to sustain appropriate livelihood, systems for transparent hiring and promotion, and mechanisms to provide appropriate oversight of discretionary decision-making. In addition, regular and timely rotation of assignments can also reduce insularity and corruption.

6.3 Health related human resource and reform

Reform of health related human resource should be appropriate to the needs of the country's health system with due attention to numerical inadequacies, issues related to mal-distribution and deployment, lack of diversity, problems with capacity building, training and regulation. The interface of human resource with other health systems restructuring domains—decentralization, out-sourcing, granting autonomy, public-private relationships—and the potential impact of reform in these areas on human resource should also be brought to bear.

A human resource policy should be developed taking all these factors into consideration. The policy should be based on an objective assessment of needs and can benefit from being translated into a *Health Services Law*, which encompasses all categories of healthcare providers and lays down consensus driven roles and prerogatives. Concomitantly, a comprehensive and consolidated *database on health related human resource* should be established to enable monitoring.

The second priority should be to *address the current shortfall* in certain categories and aim for desirable healthcare provider-population ratios benchmarking international recommendations. Such an effort should pay special attention to recruitment and retention of women in the health sector workforce. Efforts to outsource training of healthcare providers should be matched with *appropriate retention policies* and regulatory controls over migration—both within the country outside of the state system as well as overseas.

In the third place, *education, training, continuing education, and capacity building* should be reviewed for all categories of health professionals. It is also important to strengthen in-service training by institutionalizing professional self development, amongst other things. Educational and training institutions and members belonging to the teaching cadres need to be reformed in their own right. De-politicization of health educational institutions and institutional management reform can be the initial steps in this direction.

In the fourth place, the government needs to pay due attention to *appropriate deployment* and do away with the current culture of nepotism, cronyism, and patronage. With merit based hiring as a norm and with attention to appropriate placements as a priority, some of the key human resource gaps can be bridged. If this is combined with a careful assessment of administrative problems, which contribute to maldistribution, most of the current problems with staffing key governance positions and workforce can be addressed.

Finally, it must be recognized that *financial incentives* are amongst the most important influences over organizational and individual behaviour in the health sector and that issues of staff absenteeism, dual job-holding, and lack of motivation to perform can be addressed largely by creating market-compatible incentives within the state system. If this can be combined with impartial accountability and a fair performance-rewarding system, institutional and individual behaviours are bound to change.

Chapter 7

Medicines and Related Products

The domain comprising medical products, vaccines, and technologies is one of the six pillars of the health system and access to essential medicines—as interpreted by the United Nations Committee on Economic, Cultural and Social Rights—part of realizing the right to health. According to the World Health Organization (WHO), a well-functioning health system should 'ensure equitable access to essential medicines, products, vaccines, and technologies of assured quality, safety, efficacy, and cost effectiveness and their scientifically sound and cost effective use.'[314] It is well-established that essential medicines can save lives and improve health when they are available, affordable, of assured quality, and are properly used. The World Health Organization's concept of *universal access to essential medicines* and its corresponding framework for collective action outlines a number of factors as influencing access; these include sustainable financing, affordable prices, reliable health and supply systems, and rational selection and use.

Ensuring access to essential medicines is one of the most serious health systems challenges. In many ways, it is inextricably linked with the performance of other health systems domains. In view of these ramifications, this chapter should be read in conjunction with several other sections in this publication. The chapter on *Health Financing* is particularly relevant in this connection. Procurement of medicines currently accounts for a significant share of government's health spending. Medicines also account for a major proportion of out-of-pocket payments made by people in order to access healthcare. Recommendations to reform health financing in the respective chapter draw attention to the current gap in public financing of health and recommend various policy options to broaden its base and improve quality of utilization. These recommendations are directly relevant to securing access to essential medicines.

The other factor ensuring access to medicines relates to reliable service delivery systems, inclusive of supply chains. The chapter on *Service Delivery* discusses options for improving delivery of essential services through management restructuring of existing public arrangements and expanding their base by harnessing the outreach of private providers—the concept of essential services is, by definition, inclusive of the delivery of essential medicines. Various sections of the chapter on *Service Delivery*, inclusive of the discussion on management re-engineering of Primary Health Care (PHC) and hospital restructuring, therefore, have an important bearing on the objective of ensuring universal access to essential medicines. In addition, several other sections of this publication draw attention to the importance of supply chains. Procurement collusion, particularly from a broader institutional perspective, has been addressed in the chapter on *Governance*, in addition to a dedicated discussion on the subject in this chapter. The section on *Reform Outside of the Healthcare System* additionally dwells on reform of public finance management and procurement, as being central to the measures needed outside of the healthcare system in order to mainstream health systems effectiveness. The interconnectivity between several health systems domains and the dependency of access to essential medicines on effective functioning in these domains, scopes the remit of the access to medicines discussion beyond this chapter to several dimensions that have been discussed elsewhere in this publication.

This chapter is dedicated to aspects specific to medicines and related products, as inputs into the health system. Bulk of the chapter focuses on challenges in regulatory domains, as that is how existing challenges could best be described. The emphasis is on quality and price regulation. These have been used as an entry point to review the current medicines policy, legislation, regulatory arrangements, institutional capacity of the government, and issues at the public-private interface in the medicines cycle. The chapter gives a snapshot illustration of the cycle of challenges in its first section and subsequently elaborates on six of its key dimensions. Three of these relate to individual regulatory streams—quality and product regulation, price regulation, and Intellectual Property Rights regulation—whereas three others have been focused on the discussion around marketing, procurements, and rational use, respectively.

7.1 The cycle of challenges

The cycle in Figure 15 illustrates the medicines chain and the challenges that exist at various levels. Malpractices at these levels can involve both the regulators as well as the private sector and may influence any step along the chain, starting from registration and licensing to the setting of prices, marketing of drugs, and sale and procurements. These practices have a direct bearing on the performance of the health system and can reduce access to essential medicines, particularly for vulnerable groups.

The chain either begins with the import of raw material or finished products as Pakistan manufactures only a few raw materials. A specific issue here relates to the import of substandard material. At the next level in the process of manufacturing, very few manufacturers in Pakistan comply at best, only with minimal quality standards and the barest minimum current Goods Manufacturing Practices-stipulated criteria (cGMP)—both these considerations negatively impact quality. There is no FDA approved manufacturing facility in the country. Approval and registration of drugs and granting of manufacturing and marketing licenses open avenues for malpractices due to vested interests of non-*bona fide* commercial entities. These entities find compliance with regulations costly and try to influence regulators to get their products registered, speed up approval processes, get favourable prices or to have their drugs included in the formularies of various hospitals and institutions. In the area of price regulation, lack of a transparent and predictable pricing formula and the standard practice of granting price on the basis of reported price of raw material and other input-related costs and overheads creates an avenue for collusion to obtain high prices.

As illustrated in Figure 15, once manufactured, medicines are channelled through distributors or wholesalers to chemists and dispensing doctors or are provided to hospitals. Each of these steps can be fraught with many challenges. Malpractices are particularly well-institutionalized in procurements where standard mark-ups are charged as a result of collusion between public and private entities. There are also leakages and pilferages from the system at various levels. Malpractices in the chain are most evident in the area of marketing, where non-*bona fide* members of the industry collude with health providers in order

Figure 15. Malpractices in the chain of medicines and regulated products

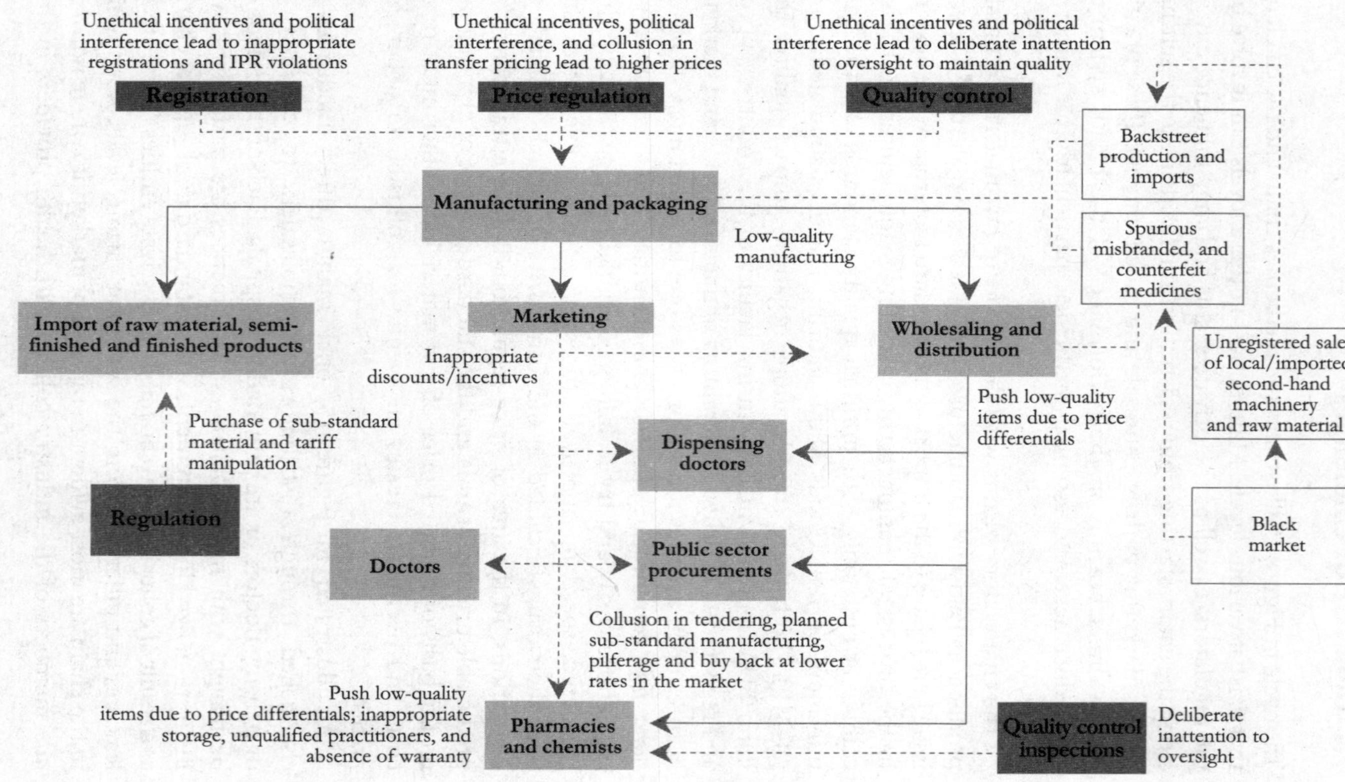

to promote the use of medicines, products, and technologies without regard for cost, quality or appropriateness of use.

In addition to the tracked and regulated sources of production and distribution, medicines also come into the chain from unregulated channels—or the black market. Pakistan's black market for medicines thrives because of its proximity with landlocked Afghanistan, which creates an opportunity for medicines supposedly *en route* to Afghanistan under transit trade agreements to be sold into the Pakistani territory, where a much larger market and hence a profit margin exists. In addition, cross-border movement of unapproved medicines is well-documented. Many a times, these are indistinguishable from licensed drugs and are sometimes sold at prices higher than those for registered medicines.

Retailers and wholesalers can also act together to create drug shortages in the market. Shortages of drugs have various causes. Some of these are genuine and may be supply and demand related such as unavailability of raw material, problems with manufacturing or decreased responsiveness of the manufacturer to low demand of a particular drug. However, shortages can also be deliberately aimed at price increase. Price differential across borders can additionally lead to drugs being smuggled out with resulting shortages in the domestic market.

All this happens in spite of the existence of the National Drug Policy and the Drug Act 1976—both are poorly implemented and are often interpreted for individual interest rather than public welfare. Issuance of Statutory Regulatory Orders (SROs) can create further opaqueness and variance in the interpretation of policies. Therefore, the first imperative—even before weaknesses of the existing drug policy and legislation are referred to—is to recognize that policies are meant to be evenly applied. Any envisaged amendment in the form of an SRO should undergo a process of deliberations with all stakeholders. Specific weaknesses of the policy and law and suggested measures to address these have been alluded to in subsequent sections of this chapter.

7.2 Product and quality regulation

Product and quality regulation covers registration of drugs, grant of manufacturing and marketing licenses, and regulation pertaining to manufacturing and retailing. This section will showcase the discussion on spurious drugs as an entry point to discuss challenges in some of these areas.

Many categories of medicines fall within the rubric of being classed as spurious or fake. These include counterfeit, misbranded, truly spurious, and adulterated medicines. Spurious medicines can get access into the medicines chain either through regulated or unregulated channels. The latter include manufacturing of spurious drugs by unlicensed manufacturers and smuggling. Both spurious as well as sub-standard medicines can also get access into the market through regulated channels. For example, when licensed manufacturers use substandard raw material and/or fail to comply with stipulated manufacturing practices, quality may be detrimentally affected. Similarly, official channels of trade can involve trade of counterfeit medicines—inadvertently or intentionally.

Spurious and counterfeit medicines are part of a multimillion dollar international drug business—6–10 per cent of all medicines distributed across national boundaries are found to be counterfeit.[315] Pakistan is known to be amongst the 13 countries of the world where manufacturing of spurious medicines has been reported. Earlier reports by the Association of Pharmaceutical Manufacturers of European Union and the US trade office alleged Pakistani markets as having 50 per cent sub-standard or spurious medicines.[316] The Ministry of Health's official reporting of the magnitude of spurious medicines in the market is in sharp contrast to this and has been reported at 0.4 per cent.[317]

The issue of spurious and sub-standard medicines is being addressed together because of the overlap of regulatory arrangements. Some of the measures being discussed hereunder, such as rules relating to warranty, market regulation of resale of raw material and machinery, and distribution chain security are primarily relevant to spurious medicines, whereas other institutional arrangements are relevant to both.

7.2.1 Statutes and their implementation

By and large, the Drug Act 1976 is a sound piece of legislation in terms of its quality of medicine covenants. However, some of its rules are exploitable. The first problem at this level relates to *warranty of drug sale* in provincial rules. According to present rules, the drug inspector allows the retailer one week to produce warranty of medicine or proof of purchase in the event of an inspection. This gives the non-*bona fide* retailer ample time to manoeuvre and produce a warranty through illicit means, if needed. There is, therefore, the need to modify provincial rules in order to make it binding on retailers to have warranties for all medicines, at all times, and for proof-of-purchase and warranty to travel with medicines. Also, by limiting the warranty to two transactions—from manufacturer to distributor to retailer—the chances of fake drugs entering the trade can be significantly reduced.

Secondly, the law makes a provision for stability studies to be conducted for all medicines. However, local manufacturers maintain that stability determined through accelerated studies conducted by the brand leader is also applicable to them. That cannot be the case because the type and quality of inactive ingredients, level of impurities, compression, mixing, and the type and quality of packing materials, which determine stability, may not necessarily be the same—brand vs. generic and generic vs. generic.

Thirdly, as the law does not mention the word 'wholesaler,' it is deemed outside of the ambit of the act. Wholesalers fall within the regulatory domain of the Executive District Officers of Health at the district level. Although they play an important role in the distribution chain, their engagement with sale and purchase outside of companies they are authorized to deal with, can facilitate spurious drugs to channel into the market. For this reason, it is important to make it binding for wholesalers to deal only with companies for which they are authorized. Additionally, renaming wholesalers as authorized distributors can bring them within the ambit of law.

Lastly, the most critical weakness in the law with reference to spurious medicines relates to its limited scope, given that herbal, 'nutritional,' and traditional medicines are not within its ambit. The currently in force, *Yunani*, *Ayurvedic* and Homeopathic Practitioners Act 1965, under which traditional and herbal medicine is dealt with in Pakistan, does not provide for regulating products. This means that 'medicines' prescribed by 130,000 registered practitioners of traditional medicine are outside of any regulatory framework. This creates a major distortion as most of the spurious allopathic medicines are marketed under the herbal medicine cover. Very often, these 'traditional' medicines also contain modern ingredients, such as vitamins and steroids—the latter being harmful if irrationally used. The *Tibb-e-Unani*, *Ayurvedic*, Homeopathic, Herbal and other Non-Allopathic Drugs Bill 2002 has been in the pipeline for over seven years now and needs promulgation as a starting point to address this critical weakness.

7.2.2 Institutional regulatory arrangements

Currently, many institutional arrangements are in place to ensure quality of medicines. At the *governance, oversight,* and *normative levels*, the Central Licensing Board, Drug Regulatory Board, and the Drug Appellate Board exist at the federal level and Quality Control Boards have been established at the provincial level, each with a dedicated mandate. The problem lies at the level of implementation. Limited capacity and paucity of resources lead to inefficiencies whereas lack of separation between policy-making, implementation, and regulatory arrangements at the institutional level, create space for manoeuvrability. The decision to create the Drug Regulatory Authority at the federal level in 2005 was envisaged to bridge this gap. However, work on that has not commenced.

At the field level, *drug inspectors* are part of an institutional arrangement, which is meant to ensure compliance with rules at several levels. Federal inspectors of manufacturing facilities can invoke manufacturing licenses. Federal and provincial drug inspectors are also mandated to exercise vigilance at the retail level in order to ensure quality at retail outlets and in the distribution chain. These arrangements are fraught with many quantitative and qualitative challenges, as a result of which there is a unanimous consensus to have greater scrutiny and higher level of regulatory vigilance in these arrangements. Recently, the number of inspectors in the field has been increased from 144 to 250, but it still remains inadequate.[318] Additionally, as systems of compensation are not adequate to sustain appropriate livelihood, corruption and malpractices are rampant. Reform to improve quality of medicines should address this issue as a priority. Systems of remuneration adequate to sustain appropriate livelihood need to be developed with due oversight. Furthermore, through partnerships between Customs and Police and ethical systems of incentive-sharing, operations can be synergized.

The third institutional arrangement includes the network of *drug-testing laboratories.* Existing arrangements are inadequate and poorly resourced. The government should invest in drug testing laboratories as a priority as these form the backbone of quality regulation. The government should also subject sale and resale of local and imported second-hand machinery to greater vigilance in order to impose an implicit curb on backstreet production facilities—the Ministry of Health should foster linkages with appropriate regulatory agencies for that purpose. In addition, the presence of qualified pharmacists at drug retail outlets should be made mandatory. In terms of timelines, however, the capacity of local institutions to train pharmacists should be brought to bear. Presently, there are over 50,000 retail outlets in Pakistan. Less than 2000 employ qualified pharmacists—as opposed to this, all the universities put together in Pakistan train less than 2000 pharmacists per year.

7.2.3 Distribution chain security

Securing the distribution chain can limit opportunities for spurious drugs to enter the medicines chain and hence the health system. Conventional methods of ensuring security within the distribution chain involve the use of track and traceability technologies and packaging protection programmes. The former includes barcodes, unique identifiers or data matrix, etc., whereas the latter can include measures such as security labels, visible and invisible authentication features, and tamper evidence. Although these technologies have evidence of impact, they are cost-intensive and require supportive infrastructure. There are additional implications for consumer education. The government, therefore, needs to explore the extent to which it is feasible to mainstream these arrangements in view of the present resource constraints.

Efforts to secure the distribution chain should also include independent evaluations and mechanisms for random batch reconciliation. These should be conducted outside the conventional channels of government inspections by an independent third party. Furthermore, drug regulatory arrangements at the federal and provincial levels should work in close collaboration with Police, Customs and other border control authorities to strengthen regulatory oversight in order to curb the well-organized smuggling routes of professional counterfeiters.

7.2.4 Pubic awareness

The Ministry of Health has budgets for and experience with behaviour change communication. However, these are predominantly utilized for preventive and promotive campaigns. There is potential within developing a campaign to create public awareness about the measures that can be taken against fake drugs at an individual level. Simple behaviour change measures such as asking for a cash memo with batch number while purchasing medicines at the point of sale and awareness-building measures in relation to the magnitude of spurious medicines and their envisaged impact can be valuable, if appropriately targeted.

7.3 Price regulation

Regulation of prices of medicines and related products is an important area of health governance. However, it is also one, which is fraught with an ironic paradox. On the one hand, essential medicines are a 'critical input into the health system' and ensuring affordability a core responsibility of the stewards of health. On the other hand, medicines are also a 'product' with considerations related to cost of production, tariffs, mark-ups, and patent protection—all of them with implications for price—operating in a market environment.

In terms of regulating prices, political and administrative attention in Pakistan has traditionally remained focused on the pharmaceutical market, without a clear separation between the *essential* and *non-essential* categories of medicines. Regulatory and structural measures in the past have included generic substitution in the 1970s, unsuccessful attempts at deregulating prices of drugs in the 1990s, and the subsequent policy of total price control, as is presently the case. The agenda of price regulation is subject to conflicting political interests and lobbying by strong interest groups in the pharmaceutical sector in an environment of weak regulation and endemic collusion. In order to achieve the objective of affordable prices of essential medicines, a review of available options is critically important.

With reference to price regulatory interventions, several measures merit consideration. First and foremost, it is critical to aim for simplicity, transparency, predictability, and affordability in the pricing formula. Absence of one or more components may either jeopardize quality, efficient supply or both to the consumer. The standard practice of granting price on the basis of reported price of raw material and other input-related costs and overheads creates an avenue for collusion to obtain high prices. Transparency is the single most important measure in price regulation in today's environment, where collusion is pervasive in the regulatory systems. Additionally, capacity should be enhanced to ensure that individual price-related components are carefully reviewed to explore where the potential exists to scale down costs. For example, whilst in most cases, basic raw material is exempt from tariff, packaging material may be under tariff, with implications for cost. In this case, it would make sense for the regulator to discourage licensing for finished products whilst encouraging local packaging, as that is how price can be optimized.

Secondly, it is prudent to explore the feasibility of implementing WHO's two key recommendations relevant to price regulation. On the one hand, these call for price control of new/branded/monopoly medicines based on their comparative performance to other medicines against the same medicine and/or prices in other countries. On the other hand, recommendations relating to generic medicines call for no price control and assume that competition will do its work. These evidence driven recommendations need to be implemented in Pakistan after a careful appraisal of their local relevance. The recommendation related to 'no price controls for generics' can usually best be applicable in countries with systems of health insurance and reimbursement, where a 'maximum reimbursement level' can be stipulated. The maximum level then becomes the minimum price and all manufacturers tend to set their price just below that level and keep it there. In Pakistan, the dynamics of medicine financing are quite different. Most of the costs are borne out-of-pocket or are paid for through government and other organizational procurement systems. In such an environment, deregulation of prices of generics is not a straightforward decision, particularly in view of the existence of a strong lobby of generic manufacturers, and weaknesses in the health regulatory system. In 1993, the impact of the Ministry of Health's decision to relinquish its authority to regulate drug prices in favour of the free market—in the absence of a mandated limit on percentage increase—with resulting unprecedented increase in prices of some medicines, is illustrative in this connection. More recently, the commodity crises influencing supply of wheat and sugar in the country point to the ability of cartels to collude with interest groups and exploit the weak governance and regulatory capacity of the government with dire consequences for the consumer, despite the existence and active intervention of the Competition Commission of Pakistan. A decision to deregulate prices of generics, therefore, has to be taken in the context of these caveats. What appears plausible is to test the feasibility of deregulating the prices of a certain set of medicines in a phased manner whilst stipulating a limit on percentage increase and assessing impact before taking decisive action.

The World Health Organization's other recommendation regarding price control of new/branded/monopoly medicines is valid. However, it must be appreciated that regulators do not have much leeway to regulate the prices of new chemical entities and that if prices are below the floor price, illegal export becomes a problem. Price adjustments according to comparative prices in neighbouring countries with similar per capita income can be a plausible option to address this potential anomaly.

Thirdly, the feasibility of eliminating duties, taxes, and tariffs on essential medicines should be explored. Successive budgets have set a precedent of this approach. However, in such cases, regulators have to have the capacity to ensure that loss of revenue is offset by gaining advantage in terms of targeting benefits to achieve equity.

Fourthly, the potential within local production and generic policies to reduce costs should be tapped to the extent possible, given the current constraints. The government should promote generic policies in line with WHO's recommendations with quality and low cost as core considerations. The key advantage of generic policies—not to be confused with the approach adopted by the Generic Drug Policy 1972 in Pakistan—is their potential to reduce cost of medicines. In Europe, prices of generics are generally in the range of 40–50 per cent below the price of the originator. The current concept of 'one-molecule-one price' being mooted by some segments within the generic industry in Pakistan, therefore, needs to be viewed in the context of prevailing global trends and logic. There are additional difficulties in implementing generic policies in Pakistan, which must be addressed. One of them is relevant to the country's local manufacturing capacity—Pakistan neither has a sophisticated upstream chemical industrial base, nor the level of needed technological sophistication. In many other countries, economics of scale and technological and industrial sophistication allow much lower costs. The other relates to issues of the post-patent era. Although these are at present, relatively insignificant for Pakistan, they will nevertheless be of some consequence over a period of time. The government must, therefore, explore innovative solutions to implement generic policies, which can make it viable for the industry to make legitimate profit while at the same time enable public agencies to procure essential medicines at favourable rates. For example, the government can select manufacturers on the basis of cGMP and other quality standards and negotiate with the manufacturer for best price through advance market commitments and bundling products. Similarly, generic policies can be implemented by incentivizing local manufacturers to produce cheaper drugs for the market, some of which are not available in the market at all. For example, manufacturers do not find it worth their while to manufacture hydrochlorothiazide—an immensely useful drug, which can make treatment of hypertension affordable for millions of individuals across the country. The government can incentivize manufacturers to produce such drugs by allowing for price adjustment and by addressing other constraints such as through allocation of adequate raw material quotas and provision of solutions for genuine manufacturing bottlenecks. Pakistan needs regulators who can negotiate prices for public interest and incentivize manufacturers to produce cheaper drugs for the consumer.

Lastly, within the regulatory domain, the concept of differential pricing should be actively promoted to increase access to essential drugs. Differential pricing is used when companies charge different prices in different markets according to purchasing power. It can allow companies that make patented drugs to recover most of the cost of research and development in richer markets, and at the same time, enables them to sell at lower prices in low-income countries. The World Health Organization actively promotes the use of many strategies and mechanisms for differential pricing. These include bilaterally-negotiated discounts, regional or global bulk purchasing, voluntary licensing with transfer of technology and compulsory licensing. Within this context,

Pakistan needs to enhance its capacity to make full use of flexibilities under the Doha Declaration on TRIPS and Public Health, as has been discussed in the section on *Intellectual Property Rights Regulation* in this chapter. Alongside promoting differential pricing, parallel export should be prohibited as this can allow exportation of cheaper medicines to richer countries, as a result of which manufacturers tend to increase their price in the country where price difference has been allowed. Parallel export can be discouraged through market segmentation—other packages, other names, etc. Global regulation can ensure that countries, which parallel export, are excluded from the price differential. This is a necessary measure to ensure that parallel exports do not kill differential pricing.

In addition to reviewing its existing approach to price regulation, the government must also enhance its capacity to explore other opportunities and implement additional measures in order to make essential medicines and related products accessible and affordable.

Use of impartial price information is important in this connection and is fundamental in obtaining the best price. Agencies must have access to reliable information as this can help them in price negotiations, locating new supply sources, and assessing the efficiency of procurement. Investments should be made to develop price surveillance and market information systems. These can ensure access to timely information and enable procurement agencies to negotiate affordable prices and make informed decisions. This is an important consideration in an environment where there are many suppliers and huge variations in price and quality. It is also important to have similar information on international transactions and procurements in order to assist with decision-making. A third party audit and its open posting in the public domain can additionally have a knock-on effect on ensuring that prices are rationalized. Tools and price information service templates developed by WHO and guidance from global price reporting mechanisms, which have been well developed in the area of antiretroviral drug supply systems, can be used as a starting point for capacity building in this area. A sustainable information system on price surveillance can also include periodic price survey methods. Such surveys can also assess factors, which influence prescribing by practitioners. Pakistan should also actively enhance the use of international drug purchase facilities to reduce cost of medicines that are bulk procured. Furthermore, it is important to invest in reliable supply systems in order to address shortages and plug leakages and pilferages from the system.

Drug donations should be actively sought as an option, where feasible. Although donations are not a replacement for sustainable medicine financing systems, they can be a temporary solution to bridge gaps in public financing. They can be particularly useful for certain disease programmes and for non-profit hospitals. The World Health Organization and allied agencies have many channels for donating drugs for tropical diseases. The use of these channels should be maximized in Pakistan.

A combination of approaches are, therefore, needed at several levels—within the ambit of price regulation and otherwise—to make cheaper and quality drugs available in the market and in the public system. Institutional factors centred on transparency, impartiality, and objectivity, which have been spotlighted in this publication in general, and effectiveness and transparency in drug regulatory arrangements, alluded to in this chapter, are critical factors in achieving this objective.

7.4 Intellectual Property Rights regulation

The importance of Intellectual Property Rights (IPR) regulation must be contextualized as a starting point. According to WHO, 85 per cent of the medicines-related mortality and morbidity occurs because of lack of access to essential medicines and only 15 per cent as a result of lack of access to medicines, which are still under patent or are not developed at all. In Pakistan, patented medicines have less than 5 per cent of the market share. As such, therefore, matters related to IPR have limited relevance in relation to access to essential medicines. This notwithstanding, since liberalization of international trade under World Trade Organization (WTO) agreements, particularly Trade Related Aspects of Intellectual Property Rights (TRIPS), can have some implications for access to drugs and their affordability, the Ministry of Health must enhance its capacity to analyze the impact of patent protection on drug prices. The World Health Organization, in its Resolution 56.27, has implied this explicitly and has reaffirmed that public health interests should be paramount, both in pharmaceutical as well as health policies.[319] The resolution has reiterated that TRIPS does not, and should not, prevent members from taking measures to protect public health and promote access to medicines for all, in accordance with the Doha Declaration on the TRIPS Agreement and Public Health.[320] The latter provides a roadmap to all the key flexibilities under the TRIPS agreement in terms of the rights of member countries. In its resolution, WHO urges countries to promulgate national legislation to make full use of these flexibilities.

Pakistan is a signatory to the WTO agreement on TRIPS and has promulgated the Patent Ordinance 2000 to comply with its requirements—the ordinance was amended in 2002. As in other countries, treatment of medicines under the law can create barriers to access, when it comes into force in 2016. Countries were meant to implement TRIPS by 2000. However, those that were not granting patents earlier, as in the case of Pakistan, were granted a five-year transitional period until January 2005, during which a mailbox facility was made available to them for receiving new patent applications. During this period, 4212 applications were received through the mailbox in Pakistan. Subsequently, there was a further 10-year extension in the transitional period for least developing countries under the Doha Declaration, which now means that Pakistan needs to be TRIPS-compliant by 2016.

A range of issues need to be addressed against this backdrop. The Drug Policy 1997 and the Drug Act 1976, both of which came into force before the WTO era, need to be updated in order to make them TRIPS-compliant. In addition, the Pakistan specific potential public health impact of TRIPS needs to be objectively analyzed. Under TRIPS, the duration of patent protection has been increased from 16 to 21 years and it is perceived that strong patent protection could mean higher prices of drugs. However, given that only 5 per cent of the pharmaceutical market in Pakistan is under patent, the envisaged impact of patent protection on drug prices needs to be objectively ascertained. The extent to which this narrows the opportunity for local manufacturers, who compete for market share of generics that are already in their maturity phase, also needs to be assessed. In any case, the research and development base of the local pharmaceutical industry needs to be supported in the post-WTO scenario, given the commitments embodied in statutes. This can be part of a much wider drive to increase investments in research and development in order to make the pharmaceutical sector more knowledge driven. The Ministry of Health has been collecting a Central Research Fund from licensed manufacturers at the rate of 1 per cent of their gross profits over several years under Section 12 of the Drug Act 1976. Recently, there have been attempts to channel these funds for research activities. This is a sizeable fund and the feasibility of using it for the stated purpose needs to be explored.

Evidence should assist the development of safeguards against any envisaged downside of the patent regime. Many measures appear plausible in this connection. These can be summarized as follows.

First, the government must enhance its capacity to make full use of flexibilities in order to override certain provisions of WTO agreements in the interest of making drugs accessible under special circumstances. These flexibilities include compulsory licensing, parallel importation, and Bolar exceptions. Article 7 of the TRIPS agreement states 'the protection and enforcement of IPRs should contribute to the promotion of technological innovation and to the transfer and dissemination of technology knowledge, in a manner conducive to social and economic welfare and to balance rights and obligations.' When this article is read in conjunction with the provision for flexibilities, its rationale becomes stronger.

Compulsory licensing, a flexibility granted under Article 31 of the TRIPS agreement, deals with temporary overriding of patents in public interest and granting license to a manufacturer who is not the patent holder. This can enable manufacture, importation, and sale of a cheaper version of a drug under certain conditions. When Pakistan starts granting new patents, it would be impossible to develop generic versions of a drug under patent without issuing a compulsory license. Under Pakistan's Patent Ordinance, 2000, the controller of patents has been empowered to issue a compulsory license. However, detailed rules and procedures for the issuance of such a license have not been developed and need to be framed. There is also the need to create stakeholder awareness about these prerogatives, given that to date, not a single application has been filed for the issuance of a compulsory license in Pakistan.

There are many examples of countries, which have successfully exercised their prerogative to grant compulsory license. Thailand's example of overriding antiretroviral patents is a case in point.[321] Other countries with capacity to export large volumes of generic drugs have additionally used this flexibility to include 'Export to countries with limited manufacturing ability' as a criteria for compulsory licensing alongside other more established criteria such as national emergency, circumstantial urgency, public non-commercial use, and anti-competitive practices. However, making use of these flexibilities necessitates both capacity as well as transparency within the regulatory system to treat these complexities even-handedly and ensure that these do not open another avenue for malpractices—the existing regulatory capacity of the government would be a challenge in this regard.

Secondly, the other flexibility under TRIPS is parallel importation. This can occur when patented medicines produced or sold abroad with the consent of the patent owner are subsequently imported into the domestic market at cheaper prices without the consent of the owner.[322] Although in theory, this strategy can allow a country to look out for the best price in the global market and import for resale without the permission of the patent holder, it is not widely favoured because it undermines differential pricing, which is a much better solution as has been described in the section on *Price regulation* in this chapter.

The third flexibility is Bolar exceptions. This allows testing to establish bio-equivalency of generic drugs before the patent expires in order to enable generic producers to market their lower priced drugs immediately after the patent expires. The drug act and policy do not cover this at all whereas the Patent Ordinance does not cover this explicitly. Additionally, implementation of this recommendation is dependent on the existence of a functioning infrastructure of bioequivalence laboratories, which is presently non-existent in the country. The Trade Policy 2008/09 signalled its intent to establish the infrastructure but the objective could not be realized.

Making use of flexibilities provided for under TRIPS is an important aspect of IPR regulation. However, other legislative measures also need to be pursued in relation to IPR. It is important to promulgate national legislation to rationalize patentability criteria and exclude trivial patents, as for example in the case of patent applications for the second medical use of a known drug—a strategy sometimes used by the industry to increase market share of off-patent medicines. Safeguards should also be built against unnecessary patenting. Certain products and technologies such as many diagnostic, therapeutic, and surgical devices, are not patentable under the law in any case. Overriding legislation should be enacted where feasible and required in national interest. The Generic Act of India, for example, creates an exception for companies that have made significant investments in generic manufacturing before 2005. The act gives them immunity from infringement suits from patent holders but binds them to pay a royalty to the patent holder. Any envisaged amendment to the act and policy must take all these factors into consideration.

7.5 Marketing

The doctor-industry relationship in Pakistan, as elsewhere in the world, is ubiquitous. The relationship falls on a spectrum. At one end, interactions range from the innocuous practices of doctors receiving drug samples and reimbursements for costs associated with professional meetings to receiving payments for speaking or enrolling patients in clinical trials. Such relationships between health providers and industry can have *some* positive effects on patient care. However, the scenario can also be otherwise. For example, doctors with 'close' ties to the industry are more inclined to prescribe a brand name despite the availability of a cheaper generic version of comparable quality. Unethical marketing practices fall at the other end of the spectrum. Under the influence of unethical incentives, doctors are commonly known to prescribe medicines without due consideration for appropriateness of need, socio-economic status of the patient or quality of medicines. The ultimate outcome of these practices is higher price and/or compromised quality.

Unethical marketing practices are endemic in many countries. However, marketing is often blatantly unethical in developing countries such as Pakistan because of weaknesses in regulatory capacity to enforce ethical standards. Examples of such practices include payments for personal items, trips and events, and cash incentives. Cash and in kind 'incentive systems' based on the number of medicines of a particular brand prescribed, have been well described. Notable doctors are sometimes 'enrolled' in such programmes and reputed chemist shops are partner to record keeping. In such arrangements, doctors who are known to have the 'power of prescription' over certain medicines, enter into 'contractual agreements' with pharmaceutical agencies. Targets stipulated in the 'contract' entail a fixed number of mutually agreed prescriptions, in lieu of which incentives are agreed upon. Some doctors are very sought-after and firms compete for contracts with doctors 'well-known' for having the capacity to deliver the desired number of prescriptions in such arrangements. Advance payments have been described to 'book' such contracts in advance. This pattern of unethical marketing is interlinked with the corporate culture of result based incentives—a marketing phenomena in some commercial circles. The minutes of marketing meetings of pharmaceutical companies and their detailed accounts—both of which are confidential as per stipulated prerogatives—can provide evidence of the nature of malpractices institutionalized in the marketing system.

In the case of high-value products and technologies with high profit margins, such as in the case of biopharmaceuticals and medical devices—coronary stents, orthopaedic implants, and other devices—the commercial sector can build a cushion for doctors in order to encourage them to use certain choices. In an attempt to maximize the size of the cushion, the commercial sector—the trader in this case—often tries to cut the intermediary out—the wholesaler and retailer—in order to maximize the doctor's incentive. Doctors can, therefore, collude with the commercial sector for mutual gains, often without due regard to evidence in decision-making.

The quest to make profits does not always move the power of choice in the doctor's direction. In another pattern of unethical promotion, the power of prescription moves away from the doctor to the retailer as that is how profit margins can be maximized. Many low-quality generic and/or spurious medicines supplied to retailers or dispensing doctors have huge price differentials with patented items and quality generics. Cushioned incentives and higher profit margins can attract chemists to push these low-quality items.

Malpractices in marketing and promotion of medical devices—therapeutic as well as diagnostic—are similar to those described for medicines. However, a further complicating factor relates to the absence of a regulatory framework for price and quality regulation and standardization. As a result of lack of oversight, the use of sub-standard therapeutic and diagnostic devices has become pervasive.

The government's regulatory system needs to take serious note of these malpractices. They need to review and analyze existing regulations, laws, and codes of marketing practices and ascertain where they need to be developed or further strengthened. They should also enhance their capacity to ensure compliance with standards and work with *bona fide* professional bodies to develop effective measures against unethical marketing and promotion.

7.6 Procurements

A significant proportion of the government's development budget earmarked for health is allocated for procuring medicines, products, and related technologies. Malpractices at this level have been widely reported. Their magnitude depends on the nature, periodicity, and size of procurements, the level of checks and balances the procuring agency has in place, and opportunities that exist for bypassing and exploiting the system.

Malpractices in public procurements can be well institutionalized despite the existence of several oversight mechanisms in public hospitals. In the case of hospitals in far-flung areas, the chances are higher because decision-making at different levels can be in the hands of the same person.

The chapter on *Governance* in its section on the *Parallel Management System* has described the well institutionalized system of generating incentives and commissions from public procurements. The volume of commissions ranges from 3–30 per cent of the total value and is dependent on a number of factors. It is also dependent on whether procurements are made from multinational or local pharmaceutical sources. Some non-*bona fide* local pharmaceutical companies offer up to 30 per cent in commission, which is indicative of their profit margin as well as the level of 'investment' they make to tip the decision-making process in their favour.

On occasions, hospital procurement staff also indirectly bypasses procurement procedures by making procurements in piecemeal consignments, each of which is below the financial ceiling authorized to the respective administrator for purchase of medicines and supplies. Procurements repeatedly made in this way also enable administrative staff to cushion incentives.

Procurement embezzlement in local purchase is another source of cushioning incentives. Local purchase is a system of hospital procurements in Pakistan that enables purchases on a day-to-day basis in the case of certain pressing needs. This system can be seamlessly transparent. However, it can also fall prey to exploitation. In the event of the latter, mark-ups can sometimes be fixed for the entire year with the supply agency, and in other cases, can be based on the actual volume of medicines and other supplies purchased over a period of time.

Administrative authorities also sometimes use local purchase as a tool to abuse the procurement channel for purchasing personal items and fancy medicines. The discrepancy in items requested vis-à-vis supplied is usually not traceable in systems because of manual record keeping. These, and other similar practices, form the basis of recommendations for institutionalization of electronic tracking systems in this publication.

Collusion in procurements can also involve planned sale of substandard drugs and selling back of medicines and supplies from hospitals back into the market. To get around the issue of pilferage, the government took a policy decision to pre-mark consignments, at one point. However, the 'system' got around this by wholesalers buying back pre-marked consignments and selling them at lower costs to the same or other hospitals. Sale of consignments to hospitals at costs that were not commercially viable was evidence of such practices.

In the case of equipment procurements, over-invoicing can create a huge margin. Blatant procurement frauds have been documented in this area. Other forms of malpractices have also emerged over time. For example, in technologically sophisticated high-budget equipment procurements, doctors tend to ask for equipment with very narrow specifications—a choice often dictated by pre-arranged incentives. Even if incentives are not in the form of outright payments or bribes, 'paybacks' in the form of sponsorships are well described, and although these may be legal, the manner in which they influence decision-making as it relates to technical advice vis-à-vis the use of state funds, raises many conflict-of-interest concerns. In such situations, higher costs can be levied with the danger that the procured item may not be the ideal one for the system.

Mainstreaming transparency in procurements is necessary in order to limit space for manoeuvrability. The chapter on *Structural Reform of the State* has outlined the importance of reform of public financial management and electronic procurement reforms as one of the measures to address current malpractices in this arena.

7.7 Rational use

The World Health Organization's conceptual framework, which aims to improve access to essential medicines, regards rational selection as one of its four pillars and states that rational selection can be pursued through three tools—national treatment guidelines, national lists of essential medicines, and their rational use. All three have been defined by WHO.

Ideally, national treatment guidelines should guide the development of a national essential drug list. The latter should then be used for procurement, reimbursement, training, donations, and supervision. Rational use of these drugs should, in turn, be ensured through a number of measures such as rational prescribing, responsible use, and due therapeutic compliance. However, there are many challenges in each area. The development of treatment guidelines has traditionally been *ad hoc* in the country and has largely been supported by the industry in many disciplines. Because of limitations in capacity and low demand, there have been very few attempts to determine locally suited management priorities and develop guidelines relevant to indigenous disease profiles and resource realities. Management guidelines developed for western high-resource settings, therefore, often remain widely in use—a model most industries tend to promote. Despite the existence of many professional associations, there has been no change in this culture over the years.

Pakistan does have a national essential drug list, which currently contains more than 400 drugs—the largest in the South Asian region. Many brands of the same molecule are included with wide price differentials causing confusion in procurement. There are many outliers in terms of usage with limited justification for their inclusion. The core purpose, which centres on the use of the essential drug list as a yardstick for several objectives mentioned previously, is therefore, not served.

Rational use, which is the third and perhaps most important pillar of rational selection, encompasses many concepts in its own right. Irrational prescribing and dispensing, self-medication, and non-compliance undermine its objectives. Irrational use manifests itself as misuse, under-use, and over-use, and can lead to escalated per capita costs or lack of access. Many factors at different levels within the health system—poor quality of care in general and lack of regulatory controls in particular—alluded to in the previous sections, contribute to irrational use. Unregulated sale of medicines, inexperienced retailers, over-the-counter sale of medicines, rampant self-medication, and substitution by unqualified staff are some of the institutional factors, amongst others that have previously been discussed. Rampant illiteracy, poverty, and lack of awareness compound these issues. The solutions to this problem are multifaceted and have been addressed at various levels in this chapter. However, additionally, consumer education and empowerment through dedicated behaviour change campaigns can play a very important role in this regard.

7.8 Medicines, related products, and reform

Medicines, products, and related technologies constitute an important input into the health system. One of the goals of the health system should, therefore, be to make quality essential medicines and technologies accessible, affordable, and consumer friendly for all and to promote their rational use in the health system. Within this context, the following imperatives underscore the need for reform in this area.

The first priority is to *review and update the National Drug Policy 1997 and the Drug Act 1976* in order to address gaps that have emerged as a result of contemporary considerations—trends in technology and advertising and WTO agreements. It is also important to review and update clauses and covenants that are exploitable with reference to product, quality and price regulation and coordinate the policy and law with trade, investment, IPR, and consumer protection policies. The scope of policy and legislation needs to be expanded to cover medical devices, related healthcare technologies, health products, and traditional medicines, which are presently outside of its remit. Capacity should be developed to enable the health sector to take advantage of country prerogatives to override certain provisions of WTO agreements in the interest of public health, as appropriate, under specific circumstances.

Secondly, it is critical to *ensure that the policy and law are implemented in their true spirit.* Reform of instruments of governance and structural processes of the state discussed in the respective chapters assume great importance in this regard. Without attention to these, isolated restructuring of policy and statutes will have limited impact. Specific to medicines and related technologies, it is most important to minimize collusion in regulation and limit space for manoeuvrability by separating the functions of policy-making, implementation, and regulation in institutional arrangements. It is also important to ensure uniform implementation of policies through transparency in governance, adequate resourcing of the regulatory system, and creation of windows for direct involvement of consumers. Other *transparency building measures* include incentivizing field regulation, adequately resourcing the drug testing infrastructure, creating public awareness, and making strategic interventions to enhance distribution chain security.

Thirdly, in tandem with efforts to promote transparency in governance, there is a need to build the *capacity of the state system for effective regulation and oversight.* Measures at the regulatory level need to be promoted in order to strengthen quality, price, and IPR regulation. It is imperative to ensure predictability and transparency in the pricing formula and mainstream innovations, as appropriate, to rationalize prices and establish price information systems in order to enable procurement agencies to make evidence based decisions. Decisions on procurements should take into account, both cost as well as quality. Additional regulatory measures to check mushrooming of spurious drugs should involve imposition of conditional bans on the resale of machinery, restrictions on the sale of raw materials in the open market, and stricter penalties for violation of the law. In the space of regulation, factors contributing to shortages of essential medicines should also be effectively addressed by removing genuine manufacturing bottlenecks and countering manufacturing monopolies. Furthermore, local regulations need to be strengthened in line with the international code of marketing practices to address hospitality-based incentive-intense marketing practices, which are currently endemic. Partnerships should be fostered with medical and professional bodies to build appropriate safeguards and to institutionalize clinical and prescription audit.

Lastly, it is important to appreciate that any effort in the health sector within the domain of medicines and related technologies should primarily be focused on making quality essential medicines affordable and accessible for all, as a priority. Any objective relevant to the business side of pharmaceuticals must be subservient to this core objective. The need to end this chapter on this note has arisen in view of statements from the government to pursue export targets in this area—an objective, which may be substantive in its own right but which is certainly not the prime objective of a health system.

Chapter 8

Technology in Health Systems

The use of technology can bring significant value to many health systems domains by improving efficiency, controlling costs, reducing human errors, facilitating new services, and improving connectivity. It can also assist with minimizing leakages and pilferages from the health system. Appropriate use of technology can help revolutionize learning, Continuing Medical Education (CME), and information dissemination.

Technology has been used in many health systems domains in Pakistan. However, most applications of note have been by the private sector and despite the enabling environment created in Pakistan in the last decade, particularly with regard to telecommunications, the potential within technology to promote equity and quality in health systems has not been fully capitalized by the public sector. Pakistan's telecommunications infrastructure compares favourably with most developing countries. In particular, mobile networks have expanded at a very rapid pace—there are over 90 million mobile phone subscribers in the country today.[323] Mobile networks can be effectively used to transfer short snippets of data, which are generally sufficient for reporting basic statistics. In addition, mobile technology can also enable information dissemination and payments—both attributes can be valuable in health systems reengineering. Broadband penetration, which was abysmal until only a couple of years ago, has seen a healthy growth, in part due to the WiMax technology. The government is also utilizing the Universal Service Fund to increase broadband penetration in under-served areas. Broadband networks are ideally suited to multimedia applications like e-learning, diagnostic data transfer, CME, and telemedicine. Existing network connectivity must be capitalized in order to introduce these applications.

The slow adoption of technology by the public sector is attributed to budgetary constraints. In addition, there is also an element of reluctance to change. It is important that the government brings to bear, the potential advantages of technology—cost control, efficiency gains, and reduction in pilferages—in priority setting and resource allocation decisions.

One of the most useful applications of technology in the health sector is in the area of *health information systems.* The relevant chapter outlines the configuration of Pakistan's health information systems and alludes to the technical and organizational gaps that exist at each level. Technology can have a specific application in each of Pakistan's many health information systems.

By and large, Pakistan's facility-based and field level data collection systems do not make optimal use of technology. The Ministry of Health has a nationwide Health Management and Information System (HMIS), which collects data from over 6000 First Level Care Facilities (FLCFs). This extensive infrastructure is paper based. Data transmission from source to the central system, therefore, takes a long time. Each district has a facility with a single computer where data from various sources is aggregated and keyed into a computer. The flow of data from the districts to the centre is not done uniformly. In some cases, it is sent as an email attachment to the respective province, whereas in other cases, removable media are used. Data is subsequently aggregated at the provincial level from where it is sent to the central HMIS, again mostly through removable media. A pilot project was previously initiated in four districts to automate the process of data collection and transmission. The outcome of the pilot and plans of scalability, if any, are not available in the public domain. With the availability of mobile devices, bar code readers, Radio Frequency Identification (RFID) technology, and broadband networks, innovative solutions for keeping data current at source, transmitting data to a central location, and collating and aggregating data within the HMIS need to be explored and appropriate actions prioritized. Availability of aggregate data from FLCFs can enable policy-makers to make informed decisions.

The HMIS is currently confined to FLCFs. The District Health Management and Information System (DHMIS), which is a pilot to improve the HMIS, additionally encompasses secondary level facilities but is only limited to four districts. By and large, therefore, public hospitals are outside of the remit of HMIS. Although e-solutions have been mainstreamed in some well-resourced settings, notably in the Fauji Foundation system and the Armed Forces health system, and hospital information systems have been deployed in some federal government hospitals, they remain isolated islands and have not been integrated with the national HMIS. At the district and *Tehsil* levels, some initiatives have been undertaken through donor-funded projects but these are a long way from having any substantial impact. A few high-end private sector hospitals have made use of information technology in patient care as well as in their administration and billing system. However, by and large smaller public facilities and ambulatory clinics in the private sector do not tend to invest in technology.

The current trend, both in the private as well as public sectors, is to develop custom HMIS applications, supported by a dedicated team of IT professionals. This model is not feasible for large-scale deployment for two reasons. First, the cost of initial hardware and software would be very high, and secondly, ongoing operations would require dedicated IT staff. Therefore, an alternative model has been recommended for district hospitals.[324] Since all district hospitals follow the same business processes, at least in a given province, there is no reason to have a custom solution developed at each location. Furthermore, given the availability of broadband service in most districts, district hospitals could link to a central computing facility rather than having their own IT infrastructure. This would provide significant economies of scale and reduce operational complexity. The software application should be developed centrally to allow access to all the participating hospitals—with each having its own data set. As broadband service further extends to smaller towns, Basic Health Units (BHUs) could also be connected to a central computing facility in a similar manner. As the district hospitals and BHUs get connected to the central facility, the infrastructure can be used for several other applications besides providing MIS services to hospitals. For instance, a digital library can be set up at the central location, each facility can have access to an electronic mail facility, electronic discussion boards can be set up, and urgent messages regarding disease outbreaks can be sent real time. These software applications can also improve modelling projections and revolutionize data management and information deliverables such as periodic reports. Both of these can be crucial in bridging the evidence-policy gap in Pakistan. The Ministry of Health must make critically needed investments in this area.

Another area within the remit of the use of technology in information systems relates to its potential use in field level data collection. The use of Personal Digital Assistants (PDAs) by field staff and surveillance workers can help save costs and minimize data entry errors. The Federal Bureau of Statistics, the Pakistan Medical Research Council and the National Institute of Population Studies conduct many field surveys on an ongoing basis. Many national public health programmes also have ongoing field surveillance activities. All of these incur significant costs. It needs to be explored if the use of technology can help in saving costs in addition to mainstreaming efficiencies. Similarly, the use of technology is critically needed in registries. Here, the main challenge is to move from paper-based to electronic systems. Low resource countries such as ours can benefit from the experience of other countries if specialized registry software is made available free of cost.

It is encouraging that the government is working towards providing broadband services in under-served areas. However, infrastructure without applications is of little benefit. It is strongly recommended that applications, like portals for district hospitals, be developed. Open Source technologies provide a low-cost alternative and can effectively be utilized for basic applications. The basic constraint in utilizing Free and Open Source Software (FOSS) is the lack of trained workforce. The government of Pakistan funded the Open Source Resource Centre and FOSS training through PSDP support.[325] These efforts can be extended by developing a core team of FOSS expertise that would form the nucleus for developing applications and proliferating this technology in Pakistan.

Telemedicine is the second notable application of technology in health systems. This is of relevance to two settings. In one, a patient based in a remote location is examined real time by a physician in a facility, which has a telemedicine link to the remote location. In the other setting, the doctor physically examines the patient but seeks the opinion of a specialist in a different location. Although telemedicine is a useful tool for remote diagnosis, there are many prerequisites for its successful application. Besides bandwidth, these include audio-visual conference facilities, diagnostic equipment that can generate and transmit digital data, trained staff at a remote location, availability of doctors at the main facility, and the necessary workflows to pull the processes together. Pilots in Pakistan have demonstrated that when these are available, telemedicine networks can be established.[326,327] The use of telemedicine was also piloted in the aftermath of the October 2005 earthquake to serve the mental health needs of the afflicted.[328,329] However, where infrastructure is not supportive, operational difficulties have been evident in pilot projects.[330] Another important issue to address in this context relates to health provider buy-in. To date, successful projects have involved doctors in pilot settings. However, for large-scale applications, sustainable incentives for doctors will have to be developed.

In the third place, technology can also play an important role in institutionalizing *Continuing Medical Education.* Pakistan does not currently have an internationally accredited CME programme for doctors. Training for non doctor healthcare providers does not conform to contemporary standards. Continuing Medical Education and e-learning can be supported by wireless loop technology, given its outreach, relatively favourable costs and high speed. The potential within rugged versions of hand-held computers and mobile phones to establish connectivity for e-learning should be explored. Pakistan's communication infrastructure can also be leveraged to facilitate *public access to information* through mobile-based community telecentres. The potential within existing pilots to be up-scaled should be carefully explored, in this regard.

Another application of technology is in the area of creating *health data repositories* and maintaining national health records. These become important as the country moves towards social health insurance and social protection as a means of health financing because of the need to precisely identify records. This is technically possible in Pakistan since two out of three requirements to develop a central health data repository are already in place—a central repository of identifiers exists in the shape of the National Database Registration Authority (NADRA) and a central repository of providers exists in the shape of records of the Pakistan Medical and Dental Council (PMDC). However, in order to meet the third requirement, Pakistan will have to comply with internationally prescribed data standards in the health sector.

The most important and least explored application of technology in health systems relates to the *promotion of transparency*. Malpractices are widely prevalent in the health system and are most pronounced in procurements and staff behaviour. Of all the transparency promoting measures discussed in the chapter on *Reform Outside of the Health Sector,* the one that appears most effective and least coercive involves the use of technology. Electronic national health accounts, public expenditure tracking procedures, equipment and supply inventories, and databases for matching staff and wage payments can assist in eliminating abuses and pilferages from the system. In addition, drug procurement reforms centred on electronic bidding can promote greater transparency in the process of procurements. Furthermore, technology can promote transparency in cash transfer systems and bring value to social protection programmes. Heartfile's recently launched Health Financing project, which has been described in the respective chapter has been launched with a view to enabling this.[331]

In summary, technology can have numerous applications in the health sector. The health community in the public and private sectors in Pakistan has experienced the use of technology in many areas. However, outside of a few examples, most of which are in the private sector, technology has not been leveraged to promote equity and quality in health systems. The health sector must capitalize on the telecommunications boom in the country to promote evidence-based, demand-driven, sustainable, and standards compliant e-health. The government must play its role by enacting appropriate legislation, defining e-health standards in consultation with various stakeholders, and establishing monitoring structures for compliance with standards. These decisions should also take into account, current evidence about preparedness of healthcare institutions to implement programmes that involve use of information and communication technology in provision and management of health services.[332]

Chapter 9

Health Information Systems

There are two main constraints in relation to the use of evidence for policy development and decision-making in Pakistan. The first is paucity of usable evidence whereas the second impediment is the culture of decision-making based on convention, personal interests, anecdotal evidence, and/or political expediency. While the determinants of the second constraint are embedded in a complex interplay of governance and overarching political factors, the first constraint can be overcome to a large extent by establishing a robust health information infrastructure.

The establishment of a robust and sustainable health information infrastructure is critical to strengthening the evidence-policy decision making cycle in Pakistan. The complexity of data sources and evidence-generating mechanisms, the myriad of sources from which data needs to be collected, absence of appropriate linkages, and paucity of efforts to consolidate evidence from different sources, compound problems with regard to the use of information for actions in the health sector. The effort initiated by Heartfile in 2006, in collaboration with the Ministry of Health and the Federal Bureau of Statistics (FBS), created a framework for strengthening Pakistan's health information systems.[333] Elements of the framework, which fall within the rubric of *data policy development,* creation of an *apex institutional arrangement,* and *strengthening the health information infrastructure* have been summarized in this chapter.

9.1 Data and evidence policy

A comprehensive policy on data, evidence, and information systems can be the entry point to fostering a culture of evidence-based decision-making. The policy should signal the importance of investing in a sustainable health information system as a priority. It should build further on existing initiatives and consolidate the country's capacity for systematic collection, consolidation, analysis, and interpretation of information and its timely mainstreaming into the decision-making process. The policy should also garner the ownership of relevant institutions. Appropriate incentives and rewards should be built in order to foster an enabling environment for research within institutions. The policy should broaden the base of budgetary and extra budgetary research funding sources for researchers in the public and private sectors in addition to supporting and strengthening institutions with research as a core mandate.

The policy should be able to mobilize the influence of networks and key stakeholders to communicate evidence and foster knowledge sharing. It should also leverage the use of technology as a priority to bridge communication gaps. In addition, it should mandate an institutional mechanism for ethical oversight of research within the country. Furthermore, it should articulate a consensus over a minimum set of indicators for Pakistan's health information system, drawing further on the set of indicators developed previously.[334]

9.2 Apex institutional arrangement

Appropriate capacity to consolidate, analyze, and interpret information is the first step towards strengthening the evidence-policy decision-making cycle—a gap at this level can be an impediment to the use of evidence in policy- and decision-making. A robust health information apex agency can play an important role in this regard by helping to overcome the currently prevailing fragmentation in various data streams.

An apex institutional arrangement within the health information system should ideally be mandated to collate, consolidate, analyze, interpret, and report data and information, and communicate it effectively for decision-making at appropriate levels within the health system. Countries have used various connotations for such arrangements, of which *information observatory* is the most popular. A health information apex agency should be able to identify national health information needs as a first step. It should be able to develop uniform standards for ensuring quality in data reporting and create an inventory of data sources relevant to the health system. It should also enable the consolidation of *ad hoc*, overlapping, or stand-alone data systems and coordinate donor driven data activities to ensure that national health information priorities are met and that national systems are strengthened. In addition, the agency should build linkages with appropriate data sources outside of the health sector and ensure regular flow of data from all relevant sources. Furthermore, it should be mandated to ensure ethical conduct in research and in the entire data and evidence system.

Some of these roles were previously meant to be performed by two agencies in Pakistan—the National Health Information Resource Centre was meant to collate information whereas the National Health Policy Unit was mandated in an analytical role. In reality, both were poorly resourced and lacked the capacity to perform these functions. The Ministry of Health should mandate apex responsibility to an agency that it should work closely with. However, the agency should have some degree of independence—an attribute deemed necessary by WHO.

9.3 Health information infrastructure

Measures to strengthen Pakistan's health information infrastructure are being discussed under the domains of (a) Surveillance, in the categories of mortality surveillance, infectious and non-communicable disease surveillance and registry-based surveillance; (b) the Health Management and Information System; (c) Surveys, and (d) Health policy and systems research (Figure 16).

9.3.1 Mortality surveillance

Pakistan's vital registration systems do not provide meaningful information on death statistics relevant to the health sector. The FBS maintains a sample surveillance system—the Pakistan Demographic Survey (PDS)—which records vital events on an annual basis. Additionally, it also provides information on causes of death. There are several limitations of these data. Cause of death attribution in PDS is not based on the International Classification of Diseases (ICD) and is not ascertained by verbal autopsy; additionally, data are collected by household interviews, as a result of which they are subject to recall bias.

Figure 16. Pakistan's Health Information Infrastructure

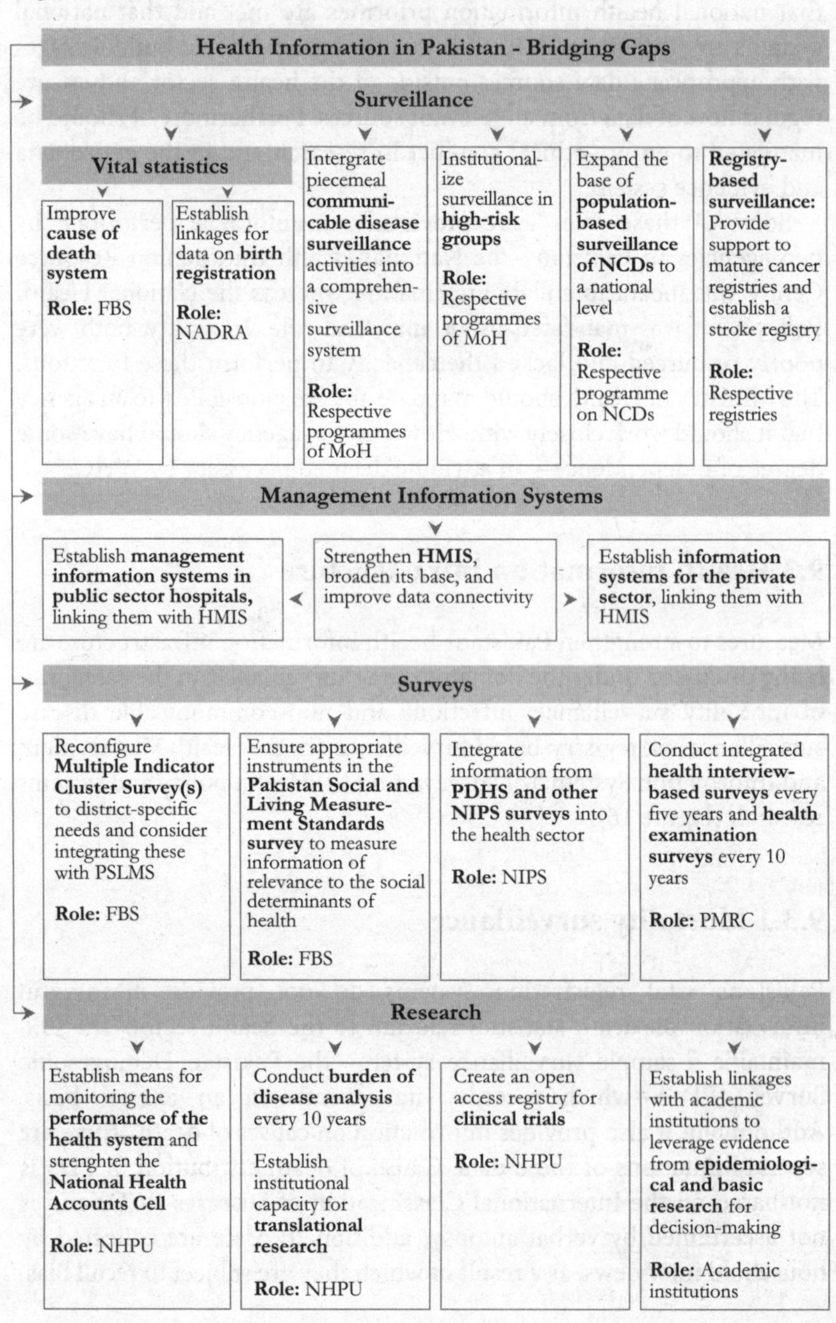

Despite these limitations, PDS can be a useful source of information regarding mortality trends if the methods and quality are consistent over time and assumes importance in the absence of other cause of death systems. Use of standardized verbal autopsy instruments and strengthening of recording and reporting of deaths by cause in hospitals can enhance the value of this surveillance system in the short to medium term. Over the long term, improvements in the quality of death records should be encouraged through appropriate policy interventions. This will require mandatory reporting of cause of death by law and inclusion of cause of death in death certificates using ICD for coding.

9.3.2 Infectious disease surveillance

Several infectious disease surveillance systems exist within individual disease specific programmes in Pakistan. The AFP/Polio Surveillance System in particular taps all possible sources of information through active surveillance methods and picks up nearly every case of polio—it is recognized as being highly sensitive. This is an active surveillance system where each case is actively searched in the community. As such, it can only be used for diseases marked for elimination or in outbreak and emergency situations. However, many of the attributes of the system, including active surveillance visits at health facilities, laboratory specimen collection, transport and laboratory testing, channels of data reporting, analysis and dissemination, use of indicators to measure surveillance quality, training and capacity building of staff etc., are also attributes of other surveillance systems. These attributes are of relevance to building capacity in the wake of the threat posed by emerging and re-emerging infections. However, the potential within the approach to consolidate infectious disease surveillance has not been fully harnessed in Pakistan.

Other currently existing channels of infectious disease surveillance—HMIS, LHW MIS and EPI MIS—have many gaps and remain fragmented. Pakistan does not effectively, therefore, have a reliable infectious disease surveillance system in place. By and large, existing systems have minimal coordination between programmes. Most of them usually do not tap into all sectors, thereby reflecting incompleteness, particularly with reference to the private sector. In addition, these systems have limited capacity to confirm clinically diagnosed cases of reportable diseases because of gaps in the public health laboratory network within the country. This is compounded by absence of legal requirements to report notifiable diseases.

A number of efforts have been made in the past to strategically analyze weaknesses and propose solutions to bridge existing gaps. A World Bank-led multi-stakeholder assessment of Pakistan's public health surveillance system conducted in 2004 made a number of valid recommendations, which are relevant even today. These called for developing a legal system to mandate notification of priority diseases, regulating laboratory practice, and integrating piecemeal surveillance activities into a comprehensive public health surveillance system consisting of peripheral data collection arms linked to a central system.[335] Similarly, through the collaborative efforts of the Pakistan Medical Research Council and the National Institute of Health (NIH), an Infectious Disease Surveillance Plan was developed in 2004.[336] These efforts need to be built upon further with attention to capacity enhancement as a priority. The Field Epidemiology and Laboratory Training Programme (FELTP) established at NIH in collaboration with the Centers for Disease Control, USA, is an important step in strengthening surveillance capacity.[337] This programme can provide epidemiological leadership to guide many surveillance systems that are currently operating independently in the country.

9.3.3 Non-communicable disease surveillance

Complexities in the diagnosis of chronic non-communicable diseases (NCDs) at the population level necessitate surveillance of risk factors rather than diseases. In contrast to communicable disease surveillance, where there is reliance on acute parameters primarily from facility sources, NCDs require greater reliance on population-based surveillance of risk factors through sequential population-based surveys, powered to detect changes in the level of risk factors, over time. This is also a valid approach in view of the fact that the timelines involved in the risk-exposure relationship also provide a window of opportunity to institute preventive interventions. In line with this approach, the National Action Plan for the Prevention and Control of Non-Communicable Diseases and Health Promotion in Pakistan developed a population-based surveillance system for NCD risk factors.[338,339] Due to resource constraints, this was limited to one district (Rawalpindi). In line with the World Bank report recommendations, the scope of NCD surveillance needs to be expanded to the national level, building further on this model.

9.3.4 Registry-based surveillance

Registry-based surveillance enables systematic collection of data on diseases with low prevalence such as cancer and stroke, through a continuous process of registration, coding, computerization, and analysis of data in a geographically defined population.

Pakistan has only a few cancer registries that conform to international standards and none for stroke registration. Although registries centred on defined populations need to be established, caution needs to be exercised as stimulating too many registries is neither feasible nor essential. It is better, by far, to have just a few that are good and conform to international standards than many that are not, and better to extrapolate to comparable populations from a good registry, than to draw inferences from a poor one on site. Within this context, the first priority should be to provide support to mature cancer registries. As a next step, the feasibility and appropriateness of setting up a stroke registry should be explored.

9.3.5 Health Management and Information System

The Health Management and Information System (HMIS) collects data from FLCFs and reports these data to the district level on a monthly basis. The system has been functional since 2000 but suffers from many limitations as a result of its limited scope and issues of connectivity. After devolution of government and decentralization of decision-making and resource management authority in 2001, efforts were made to improve HMIS and integrate it with other information systems in the country—the LHW MIS and EPI MIS. Based on the results of a study conducted by Japan International Cooperation Agency (JICA), a District Health Management and Information System (DHMIS) was, therefore, designed and is currently being implemented in four districts.[340]

The DHMIS differs from HMIS in many ways—notably in the selection of indicators and in being more comprehensive as it also captures data from secondary care public hospitals. However, DHMIS needs to be expanded further to include public sector tertiary care teaching hospitals, which are currently outside of its realm. Some of these hospitals have already established their own hospital information systems, which can be made interoperable with DHMIS. Future efforts aimed at expanding the scope of facility-based surveillance in general and DHMIS in particular should also explore the possibility of collecting data from private healthcare facilities on a sustainable basis. Currently, there is no way of gathering data from these sites. Establishment of a sustainable data collection system in private sector healthcare facilities is linked to the broader issue of regulating the private sector—an institutional change outside of the remit of the health information system. It appears feasible, however, to bridge this specific information gap through periodic surveys of private facilities and introduction of a web-based electronic reporting system for a core set of indicators.

9.3.6 Health and demographic surveys

Three state agencies currently conduct periodic population-based surveys related to health in Pakistan. The Federal Bureau of Statistics conducts the annual nationwide population-based World Bank-supported Pakistan Social and Living Standards Measurement (PSLM) survey. Additionally, it assists with the UNICEF-supported district level Multiple Indicators Cluster Surveys (MICS), which are conducted by respective provincial governments. Both gather information on a range of social sector indicators. The Pakistan Medical Research Council is mandated to conduct national interview and examination surveys—it has only conducted one to date, in 1994. In addition, the National Institute of Population Studies conducts the USAID-supported Pakistan Demographic and Health Survey. The most recent round was conducted in 2008.[341] In addition to these periodic surveys, other stand-alone surveys are also conducted from time to time.[342]

Despite the existence of institutional infrastructure and instruments, there are many technical gaps in capacity to conduct surveys and analyze data. In order to bridge these gaps, the country capacity for surveys must be consolidated. The PMRC is currently planning the second National Health Survey of Pakistan. This can be an opportunity to start building a national system for health surveys by consolidating existing instruments.

9.3.7 Health policy and systems research

Health Systems and Policy Research (HSPR) is the least developed research and information domain in Pakistan's health information system. Its definition 'knowledge that enables societies to organize themselves better for improving health outcomes' signifies that HSPR-relevant information can exist in many data streams, most of which exist in Pakistan. For example, many population-based instruments and the HMIS and DHMIS, all of which have previously been alluded to, report on indicators, which can measure performance of the health system. Tracking of in-country indicators and targets institutionalized within government instruments such as the Poverty Reduction Strategy Paper (PRSP) and Medium Term Development Framework (MTDF) can also furnish data relevant to HPSR as can operational research, feasibility studies, and impact assessments supported through budgets embedded in the national public health programmes. Databases of the healthcare industry, social enterprises, distribution channels, and retail networks exist in Pakistan but remain untapped as sources of information. Similarly, useful policy and systems relevant information can come from sources outside of the health sector; for example, from procurement, public expenditure tracking and e-governance channels, and related social sector domains. These sources of evidence have remained largely under-utilized. Efforts are currently underway at Heartfile to develop formal measures for assessing performance of the health system in Pakistan using all these data sources as part of a WHO-led Platform to Strengthen Monitoring and Analysis of Country Health Systems.

Priorities for HPSR must be carefully determined. Because of the donor driven orientation of policy-making in Pakistan, it is plausible that future allocations in HPSR are inadvertently channelled disproportionately to global priority areas. Whereas these are important areas in their own right, other locally relevant priorities must also be brought to bear. For example, one of the most pressing priorities for

Pakistan's national health research agenda should be to develop pragmatic solutions to achieve Health for All in Pakistan's Mixed Health System. While doing so, it is critical to find mitigates to the determinants, which lead to health inequities, compromise quality of service, and lead to malpractices within and pilferages from the system. This flags a number of research questions for health policy and systems research not just in the healthcare domain but also within the broader inter-sectoral remit.

National Health Accounts (NHA) is an important area of HSPR. The history of NHA in Pakistan dates back to efforts initiated by WHO EMRO in the late 1990s. The initiative could not make headway due to a number of reasons. More recently, the FBS has assumed a leadership role to collate and report National Health Accounts-related statistics. Based upon this, the Planning Commissions has decided to grant a seed allocation to establish the National Health Accounts Cell at the FBS. This budget line has been supplemented by a grant from the German government. The cell has recently published the first round of National Health Accounts. Weaknesses notwithstanding, these data are a useful contribution in the space of health policy and systems research and can be built upon further. The Ministry of Health should develop a mechanism for objectively analyzing these data and using them for policy and planning, on an ongoing basis.

9.4 Security and disease

The contemporary understanding of security scopes beyond wars, genocide, and human rights abuses to a people-centred view of security on account of the norms coined by UNDP and the Commission on Human Security.[343] In view of this understanding and as a necessary condition for national, regional, and global stability, the scope of human security in Pakistan needs to be expanded to include threats in several areas. The importance of Pakistan's multidimensional security challenges with respect to water, food, energy, environment, and health security has recently been highlighted.[344] Health security, in turn, has many dimensions in its own right, centred on epidemiological security, healthcare security and financial security, as has recently been coined.[345] This section of the publication addresses just one aspect of health security—epidemiological security—in the wake of threats from emerging and reemerging infections and public health emergencies of national and international concern; emergencies can be biological or chemical in nature and may be accidental or terrorism related. Although these are being discussed in the chapter on *Health Information* owing to the obvious relationship, it must be recognized that measures to promote epidemiological security scope beyond strengthening of surveillance and other information systems.

There is some evidence of recent increase in occurrence of emerging and reemerging infections in parts of the country. The emergence of avian influenza in the poultry belt of NWFP and the chain of transmission beginning with poultry-to-human transmission followed by probable human-to-human transmission is particularly important in this regard.[346] Virus transmission in this case was fortunately unsustained. However, entrenchment of the virus means that more human cases will occur in the future. Each initial human case gives the virus an opportunity to improve human-to-human transmission and thus develop into a pandemic strain. Pakistan must take this evidence seriously and put mechanisms in place to ensure that its public health system is capable of responding to disease outbreaks. As a signatory to the International Health Regulations (IHR) 2005, Pakistan is bound to ensure compliance with IHR stipulations and public health emergencies of national or international concern.

Prior to IHR 2005, Pakistan had some measures in place to comply with earlier International Regulations of 1968. These included a public health infrastructure for surveillance at airports, ports and ground crossings, and infectious disease surveillance. Subsequently, in the aftermath of the outbreak of avian influenza and IHR 2005, regulatory measures were introduced in the poultry sector, laboratories and isolation wards were established, and attempts were made to enhance emergency preparedness. However, many gaps still remain to be addressed. It is important to take stock of what is needed as a priority.

Foremost, it is essential to consolidate existing fragmented activities in various infectious disease surveillance streams into an integrated infectious diseases surveillance system and bridge gaps in connectivity and capacity. Federal and provincial surveillance units need to be clearly mandated and strengthened. Recommendations of a World Bank collaborative assessment conducted in 2004 in relation to the creation of a legal framework for mandatory disease notification and laboratory quality systems need to be implemented. Efforts initialized by the Ministry of Health through the creation of a national reference laboratory can by built upon further to develop a country-wide network of public health laboratories. In order to sustainably build capacity within the health system for infectious disease surveillance, training tools and methods of the currently ongoing Field Epidemiology and Laboratory Training Programme, and WHO's Disease Early Warning System can be leveraged.

Disease security systems should also link with a comprehensive incident/disaster management system as part of the state's emergency response mechanism. Issues with relief and rehabilitation in the aftermath of the earthquakes of 2005 and 2008 in Pakistan reiterate the importance of consolidating capacities and integrating institutional entities.

Policy-makers outside of the health sector must recognize the importance of paying due attention to disease security. Today's fiscally-constrained environment has placed unprecedented strains on a world that is grappling with terrorism, conflict, food and energy crises, and climate change and is unable to meet the basic needs of millions of poor across the world. In this challenging environment, the impact of a disease pandemic on the global situation could be catastrophic. Recalling the mayhem SARS and Avian Influenza caused a few years ago and the huge economic and social losses as a result thereof, can put things in perspective. Pakistan's health systems have limited ability to cope with existing health challenges even when cures and modes of prevention are known. The untoward event of a disease outbreak of an unexpected nature in the absence of vaccines or known control and prevention measures can put a crippling strain on the health system. The country must be better prepared—for the sake of its own population and as a conscientious sovereign entity, given that disease security is a matter of collective global responsibility.

9.5 Reforming health information systems

Evidence must form the basis of decision-making relevant to any area in the health sector—promotive, preventive, therapeutic, and rehabilitation and management related. It is critical to garner an unyielding political and institutional commitment to base decisions on evidence and institutionalize rational accountability of the decision-making process. Within this context, there are a number of imperatives for reforming Pakistan's existing health information infrastructure.

The first priority is to strengthen the institutional pillars of the national health information system—a sound policy, a system for ensuring ethical conduct in the data system, an apex institutional arrangement, and appropriate resources.

Secondly, it is important to develop a sustainable health information infrastructure and capacity within the health system to systematically collect, consolidate, analyze, and interpret health related data; transform it into relevant, precise, and actionable information and relay it in a timely manner for application and actions at appropriate levels. A well-resourced and independent Health Information Apex Agency must focus on integrating epidemic surveillance activities and building population and registry-based surveillance, where needed. It should also focus on bridging critical gaps in the cause of death system and the HMIS and consolidate health and demographic survey capacity within the country in order to build a national system for health surveys. Furthermore, due attention should be paid to developing methods, measures, and instruments for health systems, policy and operational research, and building and strengthening institutional mechanisms for research in academic and other relevant settings.

It must also be ensured that the capacity of the system is strengthened to comply with the stipulations of International Health Regulations 2005 and other globally binding arrangements. The data and information system should also be able to disaggregate data by socio-economic variables in order to facilitate targeting of interventions to appropriate groups—an important consideration in view of Pakistan's focus on poverty reduction as a development priority.

Part III

Health Reform in Pakistan

This section builds further on the analysis presented in Part II of this book and presents a vision for reforming Pakistan's health system. The success of reform in the healthcare system is dependent on a number of structural factors, both within as well as outside of the healthcare system. Based on this understanding, this section lays emphasis on structural reform of governance and systems of social welfare as an important adjunct to reform within the healthcare system.

Chapter 10

Reform Outside of the Healthcare System

10.1 Structural reform of the state and health

Health reform is not a sectoral phenomenon. In addition to health related policy, regulatory, institutional, and legislative dimensions, health reform is deeply interlinked with macroeconomic management, effectiveness of governance at the broader state level, and several social sector processes. These factors can have a more sustained impact on shaping health systems performance compared to isolated planning within the health sector.

Better macroeconomic management can create additional fiscal space and enable governments to spend more on health, political will permitting. This entails a number of financial sector reforms in its own right such as tax reforms to broaden the tax base, improve tax compliance, and reduce tax evasion; liberalization of trade policies to enhance exports; measures to promote foreign remittances, and legal and institutional measures to promote fiscal transparency in order to decrease pilferages from the system (Figure 17).

Structural reform of state governance can have a significant bearing on performance of the health system. The need to bring about improvements in public financial management and procurement, civil service, and audit systems, therefore, assume importance in this regard. There is a long-standing history in Pakistan of work having been initialized in many of these areas and of projects being stalled at various stages of implementation with shifting priorities as governments change. Pakistan must build further on initiatives in these areas in view of their potential to assist with systemic reform. Noteworthy projects include the Project to Improve Financial Reporting and Auditing, work of the National Commission of Government Reform, the Access to Justice Project of the Asian Development Bank, the Devolution of

Figure 17. Impact of broader governance reform on reform within the health sector

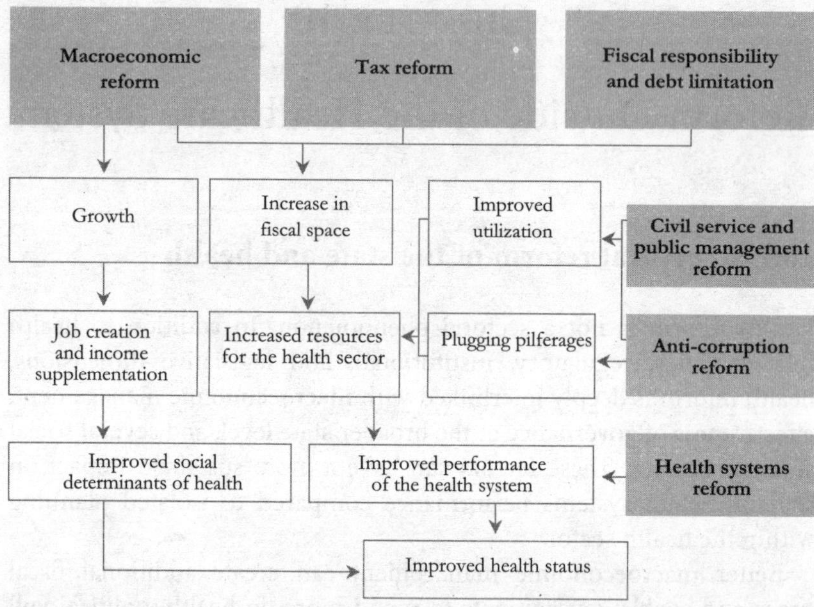

Government initiative of 2001, the e-Governance initiative, automation of the Central Board of Revenue, electronic procurement reforms, and reform initiatives of Public Service Commissions, amongst others.

The most important aspect of state reform entails promotion of transparency in order to counter the well-institutionalized patterns of corruption. Corrupt behaviours fall on a spectrum. Although it is difficult to categorize behaviours, it is useful to draw a distinction between the two forms of corruption from the point of view of the feasibility of anti-corruption reform. On one end of the spectrum are corrupt practices, which fall in the operational and administrative domains and have been discussed in the chapters on *Service Delivery* and *Medicines and Related Products*. Most of these represent individual coping strategies and are relatively more readily amenable to reform if appropriate changes are made to the incentives-performance-accountability cycle. At the other end of the spectrum, corruption involves a level of state capture, which is rooted in weak capacity of state institutions, lack of effective accountability mechanisms, and vested interests of the elite. Here, the anti-corruption agenda has to go beyond the technocratic approach focused on administrative reform to overarching structural reform that can institutionalize political, financial, and performance accountability. Reform of political institutions, strengthening systems of judicial redress and mechanisms of civil society oversight, ensuring freedom of information and an open media, and creating avenues for seeking redress become important in this connection. There is also a need to review the broader legislative agenda in order to ensure overall transparency in state governance. Attention is needed to improve criminal codes and review laws relevant to the judiciary itself. Pakistan does not have laws relevant to white collar economic sabotage and explicit whistle blower protection laws. The latter are needed to enable and encourage citizens to come forward and report on corruption incidences. In addition, it must also be recognized that economic reforms can be one of the most powerful anti-corruption strategies. By promoting competition and market entry, they can enable a vibrant sector of small and medium enterprises, which can weaken the concentration of economic interests promoting state capture. Other transparency building measures in the public sector, which centre on promoting integrity in public service and mainstreaming technology and competitiveness as entry points, have been discussed elsewhere in this book.

An anti-corruption reform is a huge agenda but if specific actions need to undertaken, they could be grouped into the following categories. First, planning strategically and reviving the dormant National Anti Corruption Strategy (NACS).[347] Many flaws in NACS have been flagged overtime. These include its orientation as an ambitious broad set of recommendations rather than the living document needed to ingrain structural reform, and its overall inspirational character removed from economic and political realities of implementation. Despite these limitations, NACS is a coherent strategic framework. It is important to develop intra-agency sub strategies based on the analysis already conducted.

Secondly, it is important to bridge gaps in institutional mechanisms relevant to anti-corruption reform. *Mechanisms of public redress* exist in the form of the Ombudsman's office but have a narrow mandate. Here, legislative action to include anti-corruption work within the institution's remit and linkages with public participation bodies such as Community Citizen Boards appears feasible. *Oversight institutions* include the Public Accounts Committee and the Auditor General Department. These need to be strengthened as tools of accountability. In relation to *investigative work*, National Accountability Bureau is currently being transformed into the Accountability Commission through an act of Parliament.[348] The new institution should be strengthened to engage in impartial pursuits. This can be done by making governance broadly representative and by fostering an open disclosure policy.

Thirdly, it is important to institutionalize integrity promoting measures in the public sector. As an initial step, it must be ensured while appointing Cabinet members that they have no conflict of interest in terms of major business involvement relating to respective ministries. This is a critical safeguard against patronage and support for debt writing off, tax exemptions, and other favours. In addition, reform measures should be used as entry point to promote integrity. The macro policy stance to separate the policy-making functions of ministries from their regulatory role and housing the latter in autonomous agencies is important in order to foster transparency in regulation. Similarly, civil service reform aimed at developing systems of compensation adequate to sustain livelihood need to be promoted. Efforts to promote integrity should also re-energize development partner efforts to promote transparency in governance as in the case of the Access to Justice Project, the Project to Improve Financial Reporting and Auditing, and other similar efforts.

In the fourth place, certain implicit transparency building measures should be prioritized. The use of technology can be helpful in this regard and can enable plugging leakages from the system, obviating unauthorized payments, and promoting transparency in procurements. Providing a level playing field for businesses and fostering competition can weaken economic interests that promote state capture. In this regard, the Competition Commission can be the entry point.

Finally, it is important to focus on disclosure and build safeguards against conflict of interest in civic action, judiciary, and political party finance. Equally important is the need to root out arbitrariness, the unchecked powers of discretion and unevenness in the application of policies in state institutions, and strengthen countervailing forces of the state—the parliament, judiciary, media, and the civil society. Whilst doing so, it should be remembered that corruption in the subordinate judiciary and politicization of the superior judiciary is well recognized; that capture of the media by vested interest groups is a potential threat, and that the civil society, which is seen as a panacea for all ills and appears altruistic may, in certain cases, has very complex motives. It is also not fair to blame the executive branch of the state entirely for the prevailing lack of transparency, as the onus of responsibility lies on all actors in the state system as well as the private sector. The latter is both a beneficiary as well as a victim of corruption, as a result of public-private collusion.

Promoting responsible governance, public accountability, and political responsibility in a system is closely interlinked with the robustness of the democratic process—many attributes of democracy are deeply interlinked with principles of good governance and transparency. However, while democracy, as understood conventionally, is a necessary condition for a good government, it is certainly not a sufficient condition. Democracy is not just about 'majority rule;' it is an amalgamation of many attributes. It is a set of institutional arrangements or constitutional devices. Under parliamentary democracy and the Constitution of Pakistan (Part III, Chapter 3), government is meant to be exercised by delegation to the executive but it is also meant to be subject to ongoing review, and checks and balances by the Parliament. In this regard, constitutional restraints upon the elected government assume great importance. Democracy is also about individual behaviour—consensus building, participation, and evidence-based decision-making are attributes of individual behaviour highly valued in public offices and ones that must be promoted as institutional norms. The other important feature of democracy is its values—democracy as a value is closely related to liberty, equality, freedom, and rights. Governments need to be democratic not just in institutional but also in a social sense with attention to individual liberties, human rights, equitable economic progress, and social justice. All these considerations within the broader remit of state governance deeply impact the performance of a health system.

10.2 Social policy reform and health

10.2.1 Social policy and health outcomes

The Commission on Social Determinants of Health has now firmly established that inequities in daily living conditions and inequitable distribution of power, money, and resources are amongst the most important determinants of health status achievement.[349] The first chapter has outlined broader issues implicit in the social determinants and factors in the inter-sectoral domain as two of the six factors determining health status. Social policy reform can, therefore, have a deep bearing on health status. The *construct of a social policy* and the *social impact of policies in other sectors* impact health outcomes through a variety of pathways, as is being described hereunder.

First, economic and social well-being are central to health. Health has a direct correlation with poverty, illiteracy, and inequities in a society. It is well established that one of the best determinants of health status achievement is the level of per capita income. This is evidenced by differentials in life expectancy across regions of the world with different levels of economic development and mortality patterns according to the level of occupational hierarchy. It is further evidenced by the observed differences in child mortality according to the income level of families and maternal level of education.[350] In many Far Eastern countries, increasing the level of female education has been the single most important factor in decreasing child mortality.[351] Pakistan suffers an inherent disadvantage in this respect with high levels of poverty and illiteracy.

Secondly, much of the scope of public health work is conventionally placed outside medical care service in any case. Provision of clean water and solid waste disposal, ensuring food security, occupational health and safety, safer working and living environments, and securing safe neighbourhoods, are important for health status achievement but are not within the remit of the health sector. The large burden of infectious disease in Pakistan is closely related to the lack of sanitation facilities and safe sources of potable water.[352] Over the age of 65 years, 14 per cent rural females suffer from obstructive pulmonary disease in Pakistan, which shows that the use of coal and biomass fuel to cook indoors is an important disease contributor.[353] The potential impact of these factors on health status underscores the need to view health in a broad inter-sectoral scope. Within Pakistan, additionally, the importance of natural disasters, climate change, ongoing crises and conflict, and the recent food and commodity crises and their impact on health should not be underestimated. These considerations additionally underscore the need to accord due attention to the inter-sectoral scope of health.

Furthermore, espousal of many other policy options outside health also have a direct bearing on health outcomes as has been described in the section below.

Thirdly, within the healthcare system itself—particularly the Mixed Health System—the role of the state in health can be reinforced if it acts inter-sectorally at several levels to ensure that health is delivered as a common good and not as the market commodity. For example, a vast majority of population in low- and middle-income countries is not fully covered for health and runs the risk of spending catastrophically. According to estimates, more than 10 million people are pushed into poverty due to catastrophic spending annually, at the global level.[354] 73.38 per cent of Pakistan's population is not covered for health. Health shocks are the commonest economic catastrophe faced by poor households in Pakistan (Figure 18).[355] Establishment of healthcare cost exemption systems in social protection arrangements can offset the risk to these populations. Furthermore, the fundamental policy shift to expand the outreach of public goods by involving non-state actors in the delivery of services in Mixed Health Systems involves decisions regarding the means of delivering social services. The decision by governments to act as payers for welfare and only partly have responsibility for direct delivery of services—a social policy decision—has important consequences for shaping a healthcare service delivery policy.

It is clear, therefore, that a focus on the health sector alone to improve health outcomes is not good enough. The potential to address these issues through comprehensive development initiatives falls within the rubric of a social policy.

10.2.2 What is a social policy?

Social policy—a part of public policy that deals with social issues—is central to politics and the affairs of the state, and is one of the major responsibilities of governments. However, while it is traditional in the public policy domain to formulate macroeconomic, foreign, and defence policies, the social policy domain often remains fragmented despite the existence of many *individual components* of the social policy fabric in the form of health, education, environment, population, and other policies and programmes, as is the case in Pakistan. Part of the reason for this

Figure 18. Prevalence of different categories of shocks (percentage of all shocks faced by households)

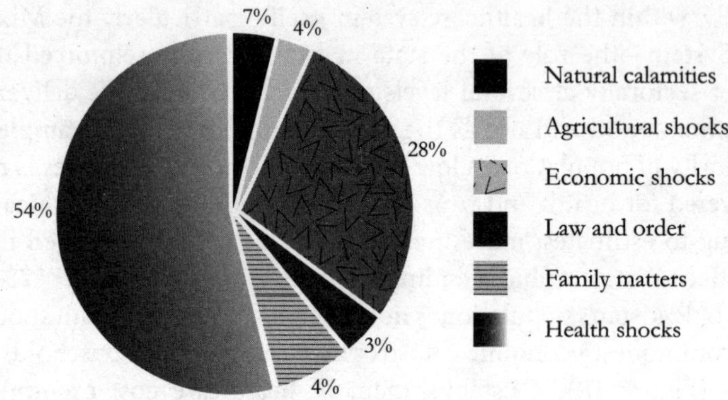

Source: Social Protection Strategy, Government of Pakistan; September 2007

stems from difficulty in housing a social policy as an *institutional entity* within a specific domain, given that a social policy is, in its truest sense, an amalgamation of policies and programmes in various sectors.

A contemporaneous social policy should encompass policy interventions, services, and programmes within the ambit of what is *traditionally regarded as being within its rubric* as outlined in Table 10, as well as take into account, the *impact of policies in other domains on social outcomes*. The former can be categorized as having four dimensions within Pakistan's context. First, a services related component, through which the state strives to deliver health, population welfare, and education services. Secondly, an infrastructure building dimension; this is perceived as being synonymous with water and sanitation. However, outside of this narrow definition, any infrastructure building effort, which assists with delivering a public good or serving the needs of disadvantaged groups or public investments in an area in which the private sector has a disincentive to operate, can be classed as a social intervention—rural roads and electrification are an example of the latter. Thirdly, as described in Table 10, income generation schemes and social protection programmes also fall within the rubric of a social policy. The latter include publicly funded safety nets and cash transfers, individual financial assistance schemes, labour market interventions, subsidies, benefits, and charities.

Table 10. The conventional domains of social policy

Areas
Services
Health
Education
Housing
Environment
Population
Infrastructure
Water and sanitation
Basic physical infrastructure
Social protection programmes
Publicly funded safety nets and cash transfers
Individual financial assistance schemes
Food support schemes
Labour welfare schemes
Subsidies on wheat and other items
Private assistance and charity
Unemployment benefits
Income
Pensions
Microcredit
Unskilled low-wage employment public schemes

The afore-mentioned are conventionally regarded as being part of a social policy. However, the impact of policies in other sectors on social outcomes is usually not factored into consideration. For example, espousal of certain policy options in the past has had a direct bearing on the delivery of health in Pakistan in terms of undermining its equity objective. The focus on export of human resource in an attempt to earn foreign direct investments has led to brain drain of critically needed workforce,[356] and efforts to promote export of generic drugs has moved the spotlight away from issues of affordability, quality, and access to essential medicines.[357] The increasing attention to medical tourism is also threatening as it can divert resources earmarked for health away from equitable interventions in an attempt to subsidize costs incurred to the private sector.[358] These considerations are becoming important as the country increasingly adopts a neo-liberal agenda, opens up its markets, and pushes the balance in the economy in the direction of public rather than private ownership. In such an environment, ensuring that the government has a redistributive role through means other than regulation and that it has the capacity to foresee the impact of, and safeguard against the negative social impact of other policies, becomes critically important.

10.2.3 Vision for a social policy

10.2.3.i Key issues

Pakistan has a range of policy instruments, which constitute the individual elements of a social policy. These include respective policies on housing, labour protection, environment, health and education. However, it does not have an over arching and consolidated social policy embodied within a social justice framework, which addresses the range of dimensions summarized in Table 10 and sets forth mitigates against the impact of policies in other sectors on social outcomes. Those in the establishment can argue against the afore-mentioned argument 'Pakistan does not have a social policy,' by referring to the Social Protection Strategy of the Ministry of Social Welfare,[359] stating that the government's obligation to chart a social policy has been fulfilled or by referring to social sector programmes and the delivery of services. A social policy is much more over arching and all-embracing than each of these. Programmes in the social sector and services are just one component of the framework. Social protection is a concept embodied within a social policy but it is not a substitute for it, and the latter is clearly more over arching. Pakistan's Social Protection Strategy is focused on 'supporting vulnerable households in managing hazards and risks'. Although it is true that the original motivation for expansion of welfare services should be to help the poor, welfare does not have to be restricted to the poor. It is now well-established that isolated anti-poverty policies have their limitations in reducing unjust social disparities, and therefore, action beyond the poor is also needed to deliver social services as a public good.

In view of all these considerations, the first imperative is to develop a *consolidated and an all-encompassing social policy* embodied in a social justice framework—a policy which includes all the elements that have been referred to earlier in this chapter while describing what a social policy means.

Secondly, it is important to mandate *overall responsibility* for implementing a coherent social policy to an organizational entity. The Social Protection Strategy of the government of Pakistan has accepted that 'there is no single organizational and institutional structure responsible for shaping, directing, and coordinating government policy on social protection.' Dedicated responsibility is essential not only to coordinate, synergize, and address current duplication but also to closely monitor and guard against the negative impact of policies in other sectors on health outcomes, as has been described previously.

Thirdly, existing issues with current social service delivery arrangements merit urgent attention. Foremost is the need to bring clarity to the *means of delivering social services.* At the normative level, the range of services and their coverage; the choices concerning those services, the means of their provision, and mechanisms of their financing need to be clearly defined. Although we speak of the state as providing services, it is possible for the state to fund services rather than directly take on responsibility for delivery. The most important role of the state lies in providing resources to pay for social services. However, when it comes to the actual provision of services, the system can be organized to harness the capacity of other stakeholders in the non-state sectors. These considerations have an important bearing on the construct of a social policy.

The government of Pakistan's individual social sector policies envisage the state as the financier and provider of social services, particularly with reference to the health sector. However, the on ground reality refutes this notion as a viable option in view of the predominance of private providers and management issues with publicly provided services. Within this context, a number of pilot projects have been homegrown over the last decade to foster participation of the private sector in restructuring the management and provision of services. Examples have been highlighted in the chapters on the *History of Health Reform* and *Service Delivery*. These implementation pilots have not been paralleled with efforts to develop normative guidance to assist with separating the functions of service financing and provision. As a result, there is lack of clarity in this domain. A clearly articulated social policy in this respect is the first step to developing explicit guidance on developing alternative modes of service delivery.

Lastly, the base of existing social protection arrangements should be broadened. This area has many dimensions in its own right as shown in Table 10. This section of the chapter will address social protection in relation to health. Pakistan's existing Social Protection Strategy includes 'protection against health shocks' in its priority areas of intervention and implicitly alludes to health in its core instruments by stating that 'the coverage of cash transfers will be expanded through *Zakat*.' However, explicit mechanisms have not been articulated. Health has also remained outside of the remit of the recently upscaled social protection programme centred on income support.[360]

Of the entire schemes listed under Social Protection in Table 10, publicly-funded safety nets—Zakat and Bait-ul-Mal—and labour welfare schemes are of relevance to the health sector. Zakat and Bait-ul-Mal have been discussed in the chapter on *Health Financing* as a means of financing social protection. Although Zakat can be a fiscally sustainable tool, its true potential has not been tapped. Bait-ul-Mal, on the other hand, is less sustainable because of its reliance on budgetary support. Additionally, the overall size of Zakat and Bait-ul-Mal remains narrow in relation to health. Furthermore, there is significant overlap, duplication, and lack of clarity in mandates. This is compounded by absence of inter-agency coordination and limitations in sharing of data on beneficiaries. Therefore, in addition to broadening the base of these pools, there is a need for a one window operation so that eligibility for assistance in safety net programmes can be ascertained, administered, and ideally delivered through a centralized agency. Gaps at the governance and administrative levels also need attention. The wide scope for patronage and abuse, discretionary use of power, and exploitability of procedures for verification, results in poor targeting as beneficiaries are selected on the basis of administratively determined criteria and identification procedures. Therefore, it is critical to enhance transparency in the use of social protection funds. Identification and selection of beneficiaries on the basis of proxy means testing, active oversight of the community, and third party validations when coupled with other transparency building measures—centred on the use of technology—can improve the effectiveness of existing programmes.

Labour related legislation in Pakistan imposes five charges on employers. These include the Workers Welfare Fund and Workers Profit Participation Fund (both of which are structured as taxes on profits); the Employees Old Age Benefit Institute (a federal government levy at 5 per cent of the wage of any person); Social Security (a provincial levy at 7 per cent of the wage of workers) and an Education Cess (a federal levy but collected and retained at the provincial level).[361] The provincial social security levy has enabled the establishment of three respective provincial Employees Social Security Institutes (ESSIs). These have provincial governing bodies and provide healthcare coverage to people secured under the scheme. Together, these register 6.89 million employees and their dependants. The ESSIs pool funds through organizational contributions and have an established network of dispensaries, hospitals, and medical facilities as is described in the first chapter of this publication.

Despite the existence of these labour welfare schemes, less than 4 per cent of the non-agricultural labour force benefits from entitlements built into labour legislation. In view of this, there is an urgent need to broaden their base. There are also many gaps in the ESSI infrastructure and system. For example, the location of hospitals is not consistent with the number of people secured, and poor governance and accountability lead to abuse, leakage of funds, and mis-targeting. In addition, the system has high costs of maintenance and low efficiency of delivering services. The ministries of health and social welfare need to work in close cooperation to bridge these gaps.

10.2.3.i Plausible options

It is important for Pakistan to develop a concerted vision for a social policy in view of the many challenges the country faces. Pakistan is the sixth most populous country in the world. More than 30 per cent of its population is below 15 years of age and more than a quarter lives below the official poverty line of US $1 a day.[362] With high levels of poverty and unemployment, this segment of the population becomes vulnerable to exploitation within the broader context of the country's current geo-political challenges. If the state's capability to target services, subsidies, and social benefits continues to erode, capture by vested interest groups will become likely. We must recognize that there are many opportunities for capture. As a society, we are deeply divided on ethnic and religious grounds; as a nation, we have a unique pattern of civil conflict and violence since the Cold War era, and as communities, we are polarized on many socio-political and foreign policy positions. In this environment, there are well-established patterns of exploitation. If governments cannot be the efficient and honest redistributive hand, the current exploitation will further deepen.[363] A sound social policy is also essential in view of the pro-market policies pursued by successive governments. While it is accepted that flexible and fair markets can lead to high levels of employment and efficiency and, therefore, opportunities benefiting the underprivileged, they can also be a source of inequities, against which mitigates must be developed.

A social policy for Pakistan is not synonymous with the creation of a welfare state. The concept of a welfare state is built on the principles of universalism; in other words, on the belief that everyone should have access to a minimum set of services. In such settings, the major responsibility of the state is to raise resources to pay for welfare on the one hand, whereas on the other, the government's administrative apparatus ensures the provision of services to citizens and processes payments based on eligibility rules for unemployment and social security benefits. These entitlements are often embodied in law, as is the case in the United Kingdom and Scandinavia.[364] Examples of welfare states include high-income countries of Western Europe, Canada, and the Gulf Cooperation Council countries. These countries typically have a high GNP per capita and the ability to earmark a substantial proportion of their total budget—generally in excess of 20 per cent—for social welfare. In addition, a majority of their workforce is in the formally employed sector, by virtue of which they also have the capacity to levy payroll taxes. Pakistan's situation is not comparable on any of these grounds.

In view of these limitations, a social policy should be approached from aspirational and pragmatic perspectives in Pakistan. Whilst it is critical to pursue welfare as a goalpost in line with the aspirational vision articulated within the Objectives Resolution of the Constitution of Pakistan over the long term, it is equally important to understand why this objective may be difficult to achieve in the short term.

It is, therefore, important to develop a pragmatic vision for a democratically rooted social policy and an operational strategy for social service delivery that is suited to Pakistan's needs and context. Such a policy should be capable of building equity safeguards in a macro-policy environment that is conceding to a neo-liberal bent. In doing so, the government must harness all possible resources of the economy towards the goal of development and fully capitalize the potential within public-private engagement.

Chapter 11

Reform within the Healthcare System

11.1 Policy reform

In Pakistan's 60-year history, two health policies have been pronounced—in 1997 and 2001. The former was pronounced by a democratic government and the latter during the period of military rule. In 1990, a draft health policy was tabled for the Cabinet's approval. This could not be enunciated as a policy because of change in government. In addition, many strategies, statutes, and statutory regulatory orders and notifications have also served as policy instruments, over the years.

The policy of 1997 encompassed many elements relevant to health systems management reengineering. A number of steps were also subsequently taken to implement those policy measures as is outlined in the section on *Decentralization* in the chapter on the *History of Health Reform*. However, these could not be taken to fruition because of change of hands on the government's reigns in 1999.

The *Agenda for Health Sector Reform*, articulated in the National Health Policy of 2001,[365] and the process of its development has been the subject of controversy since its pronouncement and has come under heavy criticism for major gaps and deficiencies—both in relation to the process of its formulation as well as its content, conceptually and programmatically. Lack of grounding in a thorough situational analysis and absence of a broad-based multi stakeholder consultative process, as an antecedent to the enunciation of the policy, have been identified as key weaknesses in terms of the process of its formulation. The policy framework additionally has a number of conceptual and programmatic gaps. These include absence of a contemporary and locally suited vision to ensure Health for All in Pakistan's health system, lack of attention to several health systems domains and health's inter-sectoral perspective, and its disconnect from burden of disease and other pressing public health imperatives.

In 2006, Heartfile's Gateway Paper,[366] and its health systems-based conceptual design inspired a new vision for health policy.[367] Based on its framework, a multi stakeholder consultation process led by the NGO was initialized.[368] Consultations deliberated on the draft of a national health policy—entitled the Gateway Health Policy Scaffold. The objectives of the scaffold have been included as a guiding framework for health in the Poverty Reduction Strategy Paper II of Pakistan.[369] The scaffold has been made available to the Ministry of Health to serve as a framework for the new health policy. Work on the latter is presently ongoing under the guidance of a task force.[370]

The Gateway Health Policy Scaffold differs from previous health policies with respect to all the four attributes that have been suggested for policy analysis—context, content, actors, and process of policy formulation.[371] In relation to *content*, the Scaffold was developed as a framework for reforming Pakistan's health systems as opposed to earlier policies, which focused preferentially on disease targets without due attention to the broader determinants, which impede progress towards achieving stipulated targets. With respect to the *actors*, the scaffold drew on a broad-based constituency of actors both within and outside of the public health system and traditional health sector to derive a consensus on the strategy proposed. The process was additionally led by the civil society and represented a rare public-private partnership in policy formulation. With respect to the *context*, the framework for health systems strengthening evolved at a time when the need for it was dire. In relation to the *process*, the Post Gateway Roundtables were recognized as a novel mechanism to mainstream the voice and contributions of the civil society and a broad range of stakeholders into the decision-making process with reference to policy formulation. The directions for reform stated in the scaffold fulfil the process criteria as they are grounded in an empirical record of the past, situational analysis and needs assessment, given that the publication of Gateway Paper II, entitled 'Health Indicators of Pakistan,' was specifically designed to serve as its situational analysis.[372]

Development of a new vision for a health policy in the scaffold was a complex process, given the diversity of health systems domains and the range of health actors and institutions that needed to be factored into consideration in the process. The complexities of health governance, multiple funding sources for health, and external drivers that impact health, further added to the challenge. The scaffold also took into account, broader structural dimensions impacting the health system—decentralization, mechanisms of social protection, labour market interventions, and health's entry points to reduce poverty. Additionally, it was also sensitive to the realities of globalization, disease security and health risks as a result thereof, the harmful effects of trade, and the aid effectiveness agenda.

The scaffold presented a vision for reforming Pakistan's health system and attempted to outline explicit directions of change at the structural, programmatic, institutional, and legislative levels. Although health systems and the inter-sectoral approach to health were at the core of its concepts, it also attempted to do justice to other analytical frameworks—economic, social, environmental, legal, and political, to the extent possible, and attempted to bring clarity to roles and responsibilities.

The scaffold envisages the following as the responsibilities of the state in relation to health:

- To ensure the delivery of essential healthcare as a public good on the principles of universal coverage;
- To ensure that people receive a clear benefit, both in terms of *health gains,* which are concerned with increase in life expectancy and reduced ill health and disability as well as *social gains,* which are concerned with broader quality of life;
- To support *poor and vulnerable households* in managing hazards and risks threatening their living standards;
- To view health within the *social sector* context as a priority and regard considerations relating to *the emergence of health as a sector within a market economy* subservient to the primary objective.

The scaffold is grounded in the following 12 principles: equity, social justice, universal coverage, fair financing, people-centred priorities, evidence-based decision-making, outcome orientation, gender mainstreaming, community empowerment, quality of care, subsidiarity, and technical and allocative efficiency. Its vision involves strengthening and organizing the health system so that it:

- Addresses social inequities and inequities in health and is fair, responsive and pro-poor;

- Supports people and communities to attain the highest possible level of health and well-being;
- Reduces excess mortality, morbidity, and disability and caregivers burden—especially in poor and marginalized populations;
- Mitigates risks to health that arise from environmental, economic, social, and behavioural causes;
- Meets the specific needs of health promotion as well as treatment, prevention, and control of diseases; and
- Is there when you need it—a health system that encourages you to have your say and ensures that your views are taken into account.

The broad goals of the new vision and envisaged Reform Agenda and their respective strategies fall within the following eight domains: evidence and information, health in all policies, health promotion, leadership and governance, health financing, service delivery, health related human resource, and medicines and related products.

The scaffold sets forth a number of alternative entry points to health related poverty reduction by embedding them in service delivery and financing reforms. These go beyond the existing focus, which is centred on addressing diseases of the poor and are focused on ensuring that public resources are used preferentially to serve the equity objective. Specific measures include prioritizing public sources of financing and prepayment mechanisms as a form of health financing rather than at the time of service expenditures; dovetailing cash transfers in exemption systems as a targeting approach to benefit the poor; reorienting government services towards the disadvantaged, and addressing neglected diseases that affect the economically productive workforce.

The scaffold has attempted to bring coherence to a diverse set of issues that need to be taken into considerations while formulating a health policy. As such, it remains a framework document and needs to be built upon further into tangible targets in planning instruments.

The original text of the Gateway Health Policy Scaffold appears as an annexure to this publication. Key directions for reform of the health system are illustrated in Figure 19.

Figure 19. Key directions for health service delivery and financing reform

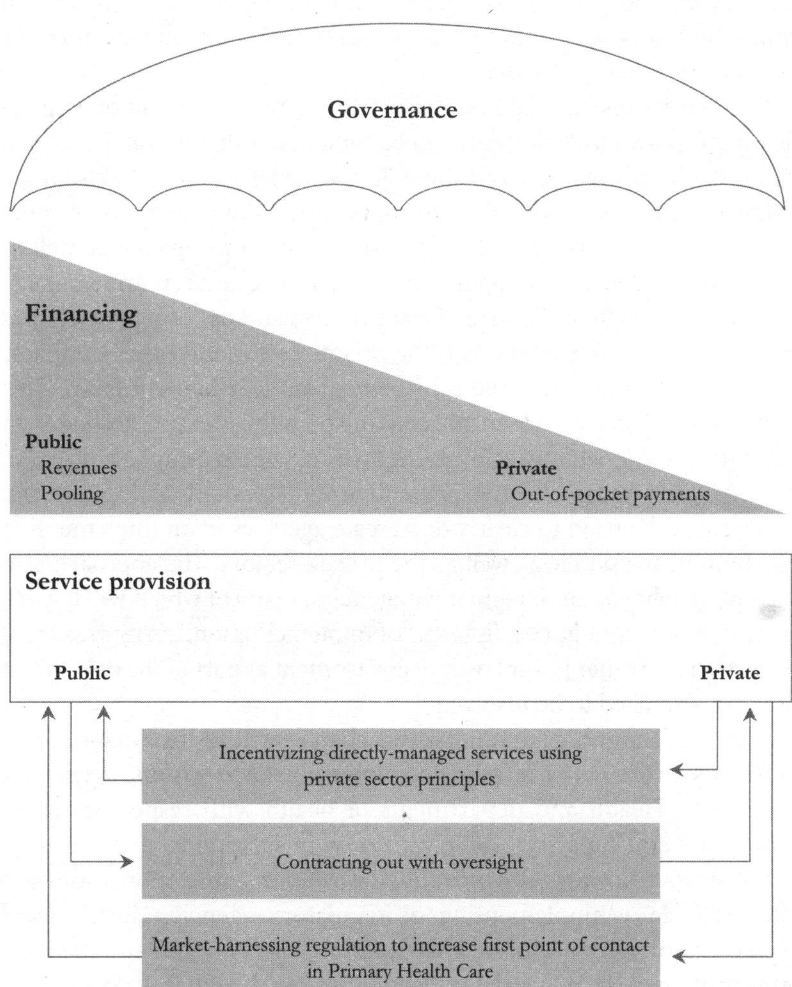

11.2 Institutional reform

Within Pakistan, agencies that are mandated in a health related role include the Federal Ministry of Health, the provincial departments of health and the offices of the Executive District Officers, Health (EDO H);

in addition, there are also a range of organizational entities in the health sector, which fall under different administrative and functional categories. Each of these has a role to play in relation to health, which is why reform within the health sector has to begin by analyzing the need for reforming these institutions of the state.

A number of considerations, of which the colonial-contemporary lag is the foremost, can underscore the need for a major institutional overhaul within the health sector. Institutions in the social sector in Pakistan are designed on a model with the assumption that the country is running a welfare state, where the role of the state is both to finance as well as deliver social services. As opposed to this, it has become an imperative to harness the strength of a range of stakeholders and develop partnerships and interface arrangements with the private sector and other non-state entities that can facilitate the achievement of development goals. This warrants a paradigm shift in the role of the public sector. It creates an imperative for enabling and strengthening stewardship agencies so that they can play an effective normative and standard-setting role and underscores the need to clearly demarcate agencies in an implementing role, both in the public as well as the private sectors. The approach also warrants a delineation of regulatory agencies, many of which will have to be created or reconfigured. In terms of implementation, current issues at the district and other lower levels of government as part of the devolution initiative also need to be resolved.

In view of these considerations, this chapter will address institutional reform with a focus on the following dimensions: *Stewardship agencies*—Ministry of Health and departments of health with respect to issues of mandate and capacity; *Decentralization* in relation to devolution of administrative powers; *Organizational entities* in connection with their potential role as implementing or regulatory agencies; institutional reorganization relevant to the *inter-sectoral scope of health* and the issue of *integration of the ministries of Population and Health* in Pakistan.

11.2.1 Ministry of Health

The Ministry of Health of the Government of Pakistan is the principal state agency at the federal level, constitutionally mandated in a number of overarching roles, which fall within the normative, planning, coordination, oversight, and regulatory realms. Although health is a provincial subject with service delivery responsibilities in the district domain, the Ministry of Health has many important roles, which are often not fully appreciated. These roles have not been clearly defined and are being over-shadowed by administrative and logistic tasks, which overwhelm functionaries within this ministry. Table 11 lists roles, which are perceived as being the core functions of the Ministry of Health, current gaps in each of these areas, and the key steps needed to bridge these gaps. It is important that the ministry divests itself from roles that lead it away from its core functions and builds its own capacity to perform key normative tasks.

Ideas have been mooted in the past to scale down the hierarchical status of the ministry and devolve controls to the provinces. Recent debates on abolishing the Concurrent List of the Constitution—this mandates both the provinces and the federation to legislate in certain areas, and therefore, legitimizes a joint prerogative for both the provincial and federal government in an area—and fully devolving health to the provincial level,[373] and NCGR's earlier recommendations,[374] which call for scaling down the Ministry of Health to a Division and placing it under a proposed Ministry of Human Development alongside population welfare, education, labour and overseas Pakistanis, are evidence of such approaches. However, implementation of such recommendations should carefully take into consideration, the strategic role of the Ministry of Health. The Concurrent List cannot be abolished in its entirety particularly with reference to the health sector. Downsizing of the Ministry of Health in the institutional hierarchy will not serve a substantial purpose and will additionally lead to an unproductive turf war. What is more important is to facilitate transformation of the ministry with attention to capacity building so that it can play an effective role in policy formulation and standard-setting, economic coordination, and ensuring compliance with international health standards with reference to health security.

As a first step towards reorganizing the Ministry of Health, a statement of purpose needs to be developed. This statement should clearly articulate the role, mission, vision, and key deliverables of the ministry and the set of outputs and processes that are needed overtime, to achieve these objectives. Capacity building in key areas and stepping back from roles that are not its mandate, must be actively pursued. In

Table 11. Roles and responsibilities of the Ministry of Health

Roles and responsibilities	Gaps	Possible solutions
Policy-making; norms and standard setting	Limited capacity at the institutional level; absence of an independent institutional entity mandated in an analytical role	Creation of a well-resourced independent institutional structure, mandated in an analytical role with strong linkages with the MoH's Planning Wing
Planning and coordination	Poorly resourced planning and coordination	Strengthening of the Planning Wing within MOH
Information and evidence, international health regulations	Absence of a health information apex agency in the MoH and fragmentation of health information streams	Consolidation of existing health information systems; creation of an apex agency, and consolidation of data flows
Public health*	Disconnect between burden of disease-related priorities and resource allocations; focus on resource management and implementation as opposed to normative functions	Redefinition of essential health services with attention to burden of disease; institutionalization of existing programmes into district accounting and accountability channels
Inter-sectoral coordination	Lack of capacity within the health sector to be effective, inter-sectorally	Strengthening of capacity to foster inter-sectoral action and mainstream health in all policies
Regulation and oversight	Weak regulatory and oversight capacity	Building institutional capacity for effective regulation and oversight
Stewardship of autonomous and attached agencies**	Undue coercive controls and limited stewardship	Relinquishing coercive controls; granting administrative and financial autonomy commensurate with function and capacity and playing an effective oversight role
Fostering transparency	Inability to address collusion in the health system	Implementing implicit transparency-building measures in the health system
Broader legislative agenda	Limited focus on substantive issues related to health systems strengthening	Focusing attention to legislate in the interest of equity and effectiveness

Roles that are not the mandate of the Ministry of Health—distracting roles	Possible solutions
Management of federal hospitals	Legislation to grant autonomy to those on provincial territory; step back oversight role in case of those in the federal territory with enhanced autonomy
Operational control of public health programmes	See * above
Operational control of autonomous and regulatory agencies	See ** above
Lack of separation between policy-making and regulatory and implementation roles	Clearly demarcating agencies in their respective roles

Figure 20. Enhancing capacity of the technical arm of the Ministry of Health

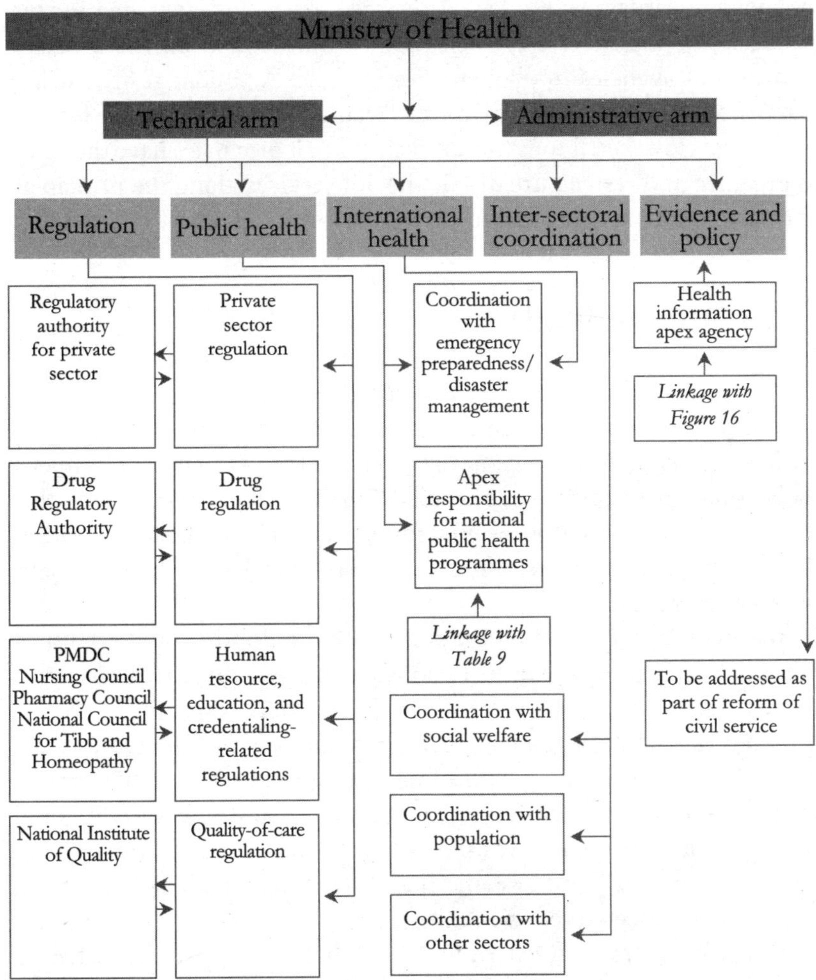

terms of enhancing capacity, the personnel deficit must be bridged as a priority. The organogram illustrated in Figure 20 proposes staffing in key technical areas with a recommendation that these be recruited on a competitive basis as a priority. In addition, the institutional culture of the ministry must also be at the heart of reform. Existing administrative bottlenecks and decision-making maladies, which undermine functioning of the ministry, must be addressed.

The departments of health at the provincial level have similar capacity limitations. Appropriate capacity at this level becomes important as we move towards new models of service delivery, as envisaged in this publication—the success of such models will depend on the capacity of oversight agencies to play an effective role. A similar restructuring plan as outlined for the Ministry of Health should be adopted for the provinces. However, it must be appreciated that provinces have the right to organize and restructure district health services along the principles of decentralization and local self-governance.

11.2.2 Decentralization

The historical perspective of decentralization, as it relates to the government system, has been discussed in chapter 1. To date, the most radical and significant decentralization reform—which also happens to be the most recent—was implemented in 2001. As part of this initiative, an integrated local government system was installed within the provincial framework through the Provincial Local Government Ordinances 2001.[375]

The main change in the new system involved reducing the level of hierarchy within the province. Previously, there were three administrative units at the district, divisional, and provincial levels, respectively. As part of decentralized arrangements, divisional and district structures were merged. The administrative and financial powers of divisional offices were, by and large, delegated to the district level, where a three tiered local government system was put in place with enhanced operational autonomy. In the new system, the district bureaucracy was made responsible to elected representatives.

The reform has suffered from many challenges over the last nine years. Many provincial decrees watered down covenants that related to decentralization of financial and administrative authority, even during the tenure of the government, which had initialized the reform. Under the new government, 2008 onwards, major changes have been introduced in Punjab and NWFP. In both the cases, changes have been made through amendments in the respective Revenue Acts since the Local Government Ordinances have been given constitutional protection under the Sixth Schedule of the Constitution until December 2009. Most recently, provincial governments have stated that they wish to abolish the system entirely. A final decision is awaited from the President of Pakistan, as only he has the right to override the constitutional bar, which prohibits the provinces from repealing or amending the law.

The provinces have the right to restructure the system according to the mandate articulated in Article 140(A) of the Constitution of Pakistan, which seeks to implement Article 32 of the Principles of Policy. However, that prerogative needs to be exercised with great prudence as scrapping something as major as the local government system without a thorough analysis may further weaken grass roots governance.

Devolution and decentralization are complex processes, which entail a range of transformations in the public sector. Effective implementation of this reform is dependent on the capacity and will of the government to implement changes in a complex environment. There were issues at both levels despite high-level commitment during the initial phase. In addition, many systemic issues, which are briefly alluded to here, posed an impediment to the reform's implementation.

First, the system was meant to replace the colonial style of command and control divisional and district administration with a style of governance where power was meant to be in the hands of elected representatives at the grass roots level. Devolution was meant to open avenues for accelerating progress in social service delivery and enhancing public sector effectiveness by bringing those responsible for delivering services, close to intended beneficiaries and making them accountable. The system was also expected to allow local voice to set priorities, encourage innovation, and improve efficiency of resource allocation. In reality, however, the performance of local governments was variable—ranging from good at one extreme to very poor on the other. Decentralization of decision-making and planning, coupled with increase in resources, worked for some districts whereas in others, the desired end points could not be achieved and the initiative fell prey to elite capture in Pakistan's feudal-dominated politics. The fact that *Nazims* were in fact *selected* to be *elected* by an assembly that they were not elected members of, was one of the most significant weakness of the system and opened avenues for patronage. This, coupled with poor application of the mechanism to hold the *Nazims* accountable, led to abuse of the system and fuelled graft. This further embittered the provincial administrations, which already alienated by the loss of administrative levers, now found that another layer of government had access to public resources. In some poorly performing districts, the dynamics of control also did not desirably change at the grass roots level and the potential within the initiative to empower citizens and strengthen the societal political culture could not be fully harnessed.

Secondly, abolition of the divisional tier exposed capacity gaps at the district level. Ideally, this gap should have been bridged through careful attention to capacity building with district empowerment as the goal. That unfortunately could not be achieved in an environment where turf battles assumed importance at a very early stage of the reform. Thirdly, the system abolished Executive Magistracy. Although the approach was in line with the constitutional provision to ensure independence of the judiciary, it created a gap at the local level, as concomitant investments were not made to bridge prevailing gaps in the judicial system.

Some conclusions can be drawn from this account. First, it must be recognized that restructuring of local governance cannot be fully successful if the central systemic issues in state functioning and political systems continue to be prevalent. Secondly, administrative restructuring should never be used as a lever to consolidate the administrative and political power base, and as a basis for controlling resources and using power for patronage. It should rather serve as a means for strengthening grass roots democracy and a mechanism for effective delivery of services. Thirdly, existing evidence points to specific weaknesses, which must be addressed. For example, the issue of strengthening accountability and capacity at multiple levels and the possibility of designing a useful divisional role, particularly with reference to technical functions, needs to be carefully taken into consideration. Similarly, there is a need to make use of the sizeable allocations for Community Citizens Boards as an instrument to empower local communities and strengthen avenues for demand side financing to support grass roots development.

In deciding the fate of the local government system, provinces should refrain from making sweeping changes and basing decisions on anecdotal reports, perceptions, and observations. The answer is not in scraping the current system and installing something *de novo* but using evidence to shape policy. Although a comparative impact evaluation of the devolution initiative was not planned at inception, data from some sources can yield meaningful evidence. The Federal Bureau of Statistics conducts the Pakistan Social and Living Standards Measurement surveys on a yearly basis. These can yield evidence relating to social outcome trends, before and after implementation of the devolution initiative. Sequential surveys of the Centre for Poverty Reduction of the Planning Commission of Pakistan can yield similar information. There is additionally a vast body of evidence in the 'pre' and 'post' studies on local revenue generation conducted by Provincial Finance Commissions. It is important to triangulate information from all these sources to assess impact on outcomes and outputs, before coming to any conclusions.

11.2.3 Organizational entities

Other than the Ministry of Health, the provincial departments of health and offices of the Executive District Officers of Health and their subordinate departments, a number of health related organizational entities, which fall within the rubric of being classed either as attached departments or autonomous agencies are also part of the state's institutional landscape in the health sector. However, most of these organizational entities are not truly autonomous in the administrative, legal, and financial sense and all are characteristically under-resourced. There is also duplication and lack of clarity with respect to their mandates and roles and responsibilities. These considerations call for reorganization of institutional structures so that roles and responsibilities are clearly outlined and the desired separation between policy-making, implementation, and regulatory prerogatives can be achieved.

Table 12 categorizes agencies according to their status and core functions, and summarizes key actions needed in each area to strengthen, reconfigure, or create institutional structures. Stewardship agencies are meant to formulate policy and provide oversight. Attached departments of the government are meant to be executive departments or the implementing arms of the Ministry of Health and the departments of health and can be mandated in service provision, quality assurance, or specific implementing roles. Autonomous agencies are envisaged to serve regulatory functions or perform service provision, research, education, and training-related roles. In order to reorganize institutional structures according to this classification, the government has to revisit the status and mandate of organizations and make appropriate changes. Institutional reorganization along these lines is a substantial undertaking

Table 12. Agencies in the health sector—institutional reform and the way forward

	Federal-level	Provincial level
Stewardship agencies		
	Reconfigure role and strengthen capacity of the Ministry of Health*	Reconfigure role and strengthen capacity of the departments of health; create better linkages with reform units where they exist
Autonomous agencies		
Regulatory agencies**		
Medicines	Establish an independent Drug Regulatory Authority	Strengthen and reconfigure provincial regulation
Devices/technologies	Develop a regulatory framework	Develop provincial regulatory frameworks
Health services	Develop a regulatory framework if service delivery role is to be retained at the federal level	Revitalize dormant health regulatory agencies and develop provincial regulatory frameworks
Human resource and medical education	Strengthen the existing regulatory framework for doctors, nurses, pharmacists, and traditional practitioners	Explore possibility of provincial regulation
Service providers	Grant administrative and financial autonomy to service providers and where possible, hand over service delivery to provincial control	Grant administrative and financial autonomy to provincial service providers
Data documentation	Grant a fully autonomous status to NIH and PMRC	Grant an autonomous status to related agencies and create better linkages with federal structures
Educational institutions	**Grant a fully autonomous status to CPSP**	**ibid**
Attached departments		
Service providers, standards and quality assessment agencies, and implementing agencies	All attached departments to have administrative autonomy; in addition, they should be well resourced and their roles should be clearly demarcated	

* Roles outlined in Table 11

** All autonomous agencies to have financial and administrative autonomy and warrants a transformational change, to which the government has to be committed. It needs to be additionally ensured that all the three categories of organizations are adequately resourced with appropriate technical, manpower and financial resources, and legal powers and authorities commensurate with their mandate.

11.2.4 Inter-sectoral scope of work

It is widely recognized that factors which determine health status range much broader than those that are within the realm of the health sector, and that modern healthcare has less of an impact on population health outcomes than socio-economic development and improvements in governance. In view of this, the section on *Social Policy Reform* in the previous chapter has stressed on the need to develop alternative policy approaches to health. Institutional dimensions of inter-sectoral collaboration at the federal, provincial, and district levels assume importance in this regard.

At the *federal* level, the Social Sector Committee of the Cabinet is the only institutional link between various ministries. However, it is too highly placed in the administrative hierarchy to be of relevance to operational decision-making, which is needed on a day-to-day basis to maximize synergies between different ministries. Recently, a Social Sector Task Force has been notified by the incumbent government; however, its mandate is not clearly defined and its structure lacks implementing prerogatives. There is presently no effective inter-sectoral coordinating mechanism between ministries, ministers, and secretaries at the federal level. A plausible option—recommended by the National Commission for Government Reform—is to mandate the office of the Cabinet Secretary in that role. A coordinating mechanism, initialized through this office, can link health with many other sectors for specific reasons. These include transport (injury prevention); agriculture (food security, crop substitution, and agro-industrial diversification—the latter in the context of tobacco control); Central Board of Revenue (taxation and dependence on revenues generated from tobacco); trade and commerce (post-WTO concerns and counterfeiting of medicines); Industries and Environment (National Environmental Quality Standards); and Narcotics Control Division (substance abuse).

Each of these areas has an important role in ensuring positive health outcomes.

At the *provincial* level, coordination exists at the level of the office of the Chief Secretary and a further strengthening of that is needed. A specific requirement both at the federal and provincial levels is to synchronize health with social welfare to bridge the current gap in institutionalizing cash transfers for health. Pending creation of a duly empowered Ministry of Social Protection, which has been recommended by the NCGR, a Health Social Welfare Inter-Sectoral Coordination Committee can be constituted with representation from both ministries and the civil society. This committee should be mandated to create and maximize operational linkages between health and the social welfare sectors.

At the *district* level, a number of coordinating arrangements exist at various levels. It is important to consolidate coordination so that a unified arrangement can be made responsible for a number of functions at the district level. Recently, the creation of multidisciplinary District Health Boards has been recommended. These can be mandated in an oversight role to plan, guide, oversee, and coordinate strategic work plans; provide a point of contact for stakeholders in the health and population sectors, and coordinate public and private roles for the delivery of healthcare. They can additionally guide decisions on contracting out services, review and critically analyze district level data, and liaise and negotiate with federal and provincial governments for resource allocations from development budgets. However, decisions on creating structures for district and sub-district coordination should be locally suited and must actively garner the participation of local communities in order to be successful.

11.2.5 Population and health integration

Pakistan is the only country in the world where *health* and *population* exist as separate ministries. On one hand, this can be viewed positively as it gives population planning a concerted institutional focus—Pakistan's population growth rate of 1.8 per cent per annum and total fertility rate of 4.1 children per woman is unacceptably high.[376] However, on the other hand, it creates issues due to lack of integrated services. Family planning is not viewed as a health intervention in many rural and urban underprivileged areas and is culturally and socially stigmatized. The provision of health, on the other hand, is regarded socially esteemed. It is, therefore, perceived that if population planning is provided through a recognized health service delivery network, the programme would be more successful. The question of merging the two ministries, and as a corollary, their respective departments in the provinces, has been a fundamental question in social sector institutional restructuring in Pakistan. There has also been one unsuccessful attempt at merger in 2001.

Recently, Heartfile conducted a qualitative study to analyze if merger is a viable option and to explore a way forward to bridge the current population-health institutional disconnect in Pakistan.[377] The study acknowledged that there could be many arguments in support of merger of the two institutional entities. These include the recent conditionality stipulated by the International Monetary Fund to scale down establishment costs and merge duplicating structures; the current emphasis on comprehensive reproductive health; recent efforts to improve returns on spending in view of Pakistan's macroeconomic downturn and fiscal space constraints; and poor service delivery performance of both the ministries, which creates an imperative for merging service delivery functions of both the ministries in any new service delivery arrangement. Notwithstanding, the study also pointed out many operational challenges that merger could be faced with. Different sources of funding, fund flows, controls, and hierarchical relationships assume importance in this regard. A historical review of efforts to date, additionally revealed that there is reluctance on part of both the institutional hierarchies to merge.

The study also analyzed how critical merger/functional integration could be to achieving desired outcomes in the health and population sectors and concluded by stating that merger is just one aspect of many institutional changes that are needed to reform service delivery arrangements. It further stated that unless Pakistan makes improvements in other more important areas, such as performance of the health system as a whole, social conditions, literacy rate, social mobilization, and women's empowerment, quantum leaps in improving reproductive health outcomes would not be possible.

The analysis concluded by presenting long- and short-term solutions to the problem. The sustainable long-term solution centred on deep-rooted reform at several levels in both the institutional hierarchies with transformation of the role of stewardship agencies and reengineering of service delivery arrangements as its hallmarks. The short to medium term strategies proposed in the paper centred on a range of specific collaborative measures with a view to building capacity for the broader systems transformation.

11.3 Legislative reform

The vision for reforming Pakistan's health system outlined in this publication and the policy and institutional transformation needed to implement that vision necessitates changes in many instruments of governance—including statutes. However, since legislation in health has traditionally been used in Pakistan as a tool to create new institutions and define human resource prerogatives, its reconfiguration to place a greater emphasis on equity in outcomes and better performance of the health system would entail changing mindsets and institutional culture—in other words, reforming the legislative agenda. This chapter will discuss the latter under four categories—overarching laws that can reflect the state's commitment to deliver health services, laws that are relevant to health systems functioning, laws related to public health, and medical liability related laws. This section will provide a snapshot of each with a view to outlining key gaps and will put forward suggestions for a way forward. Specific aspects of legislation have been discussed in relevant sections throughout this publication and must be referred to, as needed.

11.3.1 Overarching health legislation

Pakistan does not have overarching legislation in health. Although it is not conventional to legislate in this area, many countries have nonetheless promulgated overarching statues. The need to explore the feasibility of promulgating a National Health Act in Pakistan becomes relevant in view of the currently prevailing ambiguities in relation to administrative roles, responsibilities, and prerogatives in a decentralized health system and paucity of guidance on public-private relationships. Overarching legislation can provide a framework for structuring institutional prerogatives and responsibilities in service delivery. It can also stipulate the norms of public health safeguards and standards, and can be the basis of cooperation and shared responsibility between the public and non-state actors in the health sector.

11.3.2 Public health legislation

Public health legislation can relate to individual behaviours, the society, or to safeguards and standards. The latter are relevant to water, sanitation, waste disposal, accident and injury, medical patents, epidemics, and other areas that need to be regulated and controlled in order to protect health interests.

The history of public health legislation in Pakistan dates back to 1802 when the first health related law was enacted in the Indo-Pak sub-continent to initiate vaccination. In 1944, the Central Government of India enacted the Public Health (Emergency Provisions) Ordinance. This remains in force in Pakistan to date and has been adopted by the provinces as the overarching framework for many standards and safeguards in public health. In addition, a number of other public health laws have also been enacted in Pakistan over the years. Notable amongst these are the Mental Health Ordinance 2001, Punjab Transfusion of Safe Blood (Amendment) Ordinance 2001, Prohibition of Smoking and Protection of Non-Smokers Health Ordinance 2002, Protection of Breastfeeding and Child Nutrition Ordinance 2002, and the Human Organs and Tissues Ordinance 2007. The latter has recently lapsed, as it could not be ratified through an act of the Parliament. The first priority should be to review existing laws, take stock of critical gaps, and provide technical inputs to address weaknesses. Legislation also needs to be promulgated in areas where public health laws are non-existent such as in the case of health promotion—appropriate statutes are needed to create supportive environments and strengthen community action in compliance with the Ottawa Charter, to which Pakistan is a signatory.[378]

Pakistan has additional responsibilities in public health after the coming into force of the World Health Organization's International

Health Regulations in 2007—the world's first legally binding agreement in the fight against public health emergencies of national and international concern. In addition to strengthening institutional implementing arrangements to comply with its stipulations, Pakistan will also have to update relevant legislation. A specific gap in this connection relates to legal requirements to report notifiable diseases, as has been discussed in the chapter on *Health Information Systems*.

Efforts to streamline public health legislation in Pakistan must also take into account, current confusion about prerogatives of various levels of government in this area. Public health legislation in Pakistan is controlled by Article 142(c) of the Constitution. According to this article, only the provincial legislature is competent to make laws with respect to any matter not contained in the Federal or the Concurrent Legislative List. A review of the two lists shows that the item 'public health' is not mentioned in either. This means that only the provinces are constitutionally competent to legislate on this subject. Changes to the constitution might be necessary in this area in the future, in view of considerations related to disease security.

11.3.3 Health systems legislation

Legislation of relevance to health systems can relate to governance, service delivery, health financing, human resource, health information systems, and medicines and related products. Table 13 outlines existing legislation in the health systems arena in Pakistan and indicates areas where further statutes need to be enacted.

Improving *governance* in health and reconfiguring the stewardship role of the government is one of the most important factors in improving health systems performance. Recommendations on institutional reform in this publication have many implications for enacting legislation, such as in the case of establishing the National Executive Services and creating/reconfiguring appropriate regulatory agencies. In many areas, legislation can be the entry point to institutional reform.

Existing laws in the area of *service delivery* have largely been promulgated to establish state institutions and outline prerogatives and privileges of workforce. Legislative bodies have neither focused on enacting laws to maximize effectiveness of service delivery nor broaden

Table 13. Health legislation in Pakistan–current statutes and gaps

Overarching health legislation
A National Health Act does not exist
Governance and administration
The Local Government Ordinance 2001
Legislation needs to be enacted in line with directions articulated in the section on Institutional Reform
Service delivery
Institutional laws
Punjab Medical and Health Institutions Act 2003 (last updated on 14 June 2003)
University of Health Sciences Ordinance 2002 (last updated on 6 December 2003)
Punjab Health Foundation Act 1992 (last updated on 6 December 2003)
Medical Colleges (Governing Bodies) (Punjab Repeal) Ordinance 1970 (last updated on 6 December 2003)
Punjab Health Foundation (Amendment) Act 1995
Pakistan Institute of Medical Sciences Ordinance 1995
NWFP Health Foundation Act 1995
Balochistan Health Foundation Act 1994
National Institute of Health Ordinance 1980
National Institute of Cardiovascular Diseases (Administration) Ordinance 1979
Public-Private Partnership laws do not exist
Regulation
Pakistan Standards and Quality Control Authority Act 1996
Medical and Dental Degrees Ordinance 1982
Pakistan Nursing Council Act 1973
Pharmacy Act 1967
Allopathic System (Prevention of Misuse) Ordinance 1962
Pakistan Medical and Dental Council Ordinance 1962
Allopathic System Ordinance 1962
Pakistan Standards Institution Ordinance 1961
Drugs and pharmaceuticals
Drug Act 1976
Health financing
Fiscal Responsibility and Debt Limitation Act 2005
Provincial Employees Social Security Ordinance 1965 (last updated on 6 December 2003)
Charitable Funds Act 1953
Charitable Endowments Act 1890
Equity and health insurance laws do not exist
Public health
Public Health (Emergency Provisions) Ordinance 1944 (last updated on 6 December 2003)

Continued...

Table 13. Continued...

Vaccination
West Pakistan Vaccination Ordinance 1958
West Pakistan Epidemic Diseases Act 1958
North-West Frontier Province Vaccination Law (Amendment) Act 1947
Punjab Vaccination Law Amendment Act 1929
Punjab Vaccination Law Amendment Act 1925
Sindh Vaccination Act 1892
Vaccination Act 1880
Tobacco legislation
Prohibition of Smoking and Protection of Non-Smokers Health Ordinance 2002
Cigarette (printing of warning/amendment) Ordinance 1980
Cigarettes (printing of warning) Ordinance 1979
Punjab Prohibition of Smoking in Cinema Houses Ordinance 1960
West Pakistan Juvenile Smoking Ordinance 1959
Tobacco Vend Act 1958
Consumer protection
Punjab Consumer Protection Act 2005
North-West Frontier Province Consumer Protection Act 1997
Islamabad Consumer Protection Act 1995
Mental health
Pakistan Mental Health Ordinance 2001
Lunacy Act 1912
Occupational health and safety
Occupational Health and Safety Ordinance 2001
Road safety and injury prevention
Prohibition of Dangerous Kite Flying Ordinance 2001
National Highway Safety Ordinance 2000
Motor Vehicle Ordinance 1965
West Pakistan Highways Ordinance 1959
Blood transfusion
Balochistan Transfusion of Safe Blood Act 2004
Islamabad Transfusion of Safe Blood Ordinance 2002
Punjab Transfusion of Safe Blood (Amendment) Ordinance 2001
Punjab Transfusion of Safe Blood Ordinance 1999
Sindh Transfusion of Safe Blood Act 1997
Food safety
Punjab Pure Food Ordinance 1960 (last updated on 6 December 2003)
Hydrogenated Vegetable Oil Industry (Control and Development) Act 1973
Cantonments Pure Food Act 1966
West Pakistan Pure Food Ordinance 1960
West Pakistan Foodstuff Control Act 1958

Continued...

Table 13. Continued...

Environmental protection
Pakistan Environmental Protection Act 1997
Breastfeeding
Protection of Breastfeeding and Child Nutrition 2002
Disease specific public health laws
Transplantation of Human Organs and Tissues Bill 2007 (lapsed)
Malaria Eradication Board Ordinance 1961

its scope. With reference to the latter, provincial governments have engaged in various reform pilots to restructure management of FLCFs by involving private sector entities over the last decade. However, the norms and parameters of public-private engagement have not been outlined in statutes. A related development in Punjab has involved drafting of a bill—the Punjab Private Participation in Infrastructure Development Act 2003. The draft bill, which has been pending review for over six years now, is primarily relevant to the private sector's role in building infrastructure in the province, and as such, does not include all the dimensions of public-private engagement of relevance to contractual relationships in delivering welfare services.[379] There is, therefore, a need for a holistic approach to legislation in the area of public-private engagement so that state agencies can leverage all channels of health service outreach for delivering services. Other notable draft bills in the pipeline include the Disposal of Hazardous Waste Bill 2008, the Medical Devices Act 2008, and the PMDC Ordinance Amendment Bill 2008.

Legislation to regulate medical devices is urgently needed in the country, as this sector has been completely unregulated. This has been described in the chapter on *Medicines and Related Products*. The same chapter has outlined some of the key weaknesses of the Drug Act 1976, which must be addressed as a priority. In the area *of human resource*, the need to revise PMDC statute and the Pakistan Nursing Council Act stand out as priorities. The former in relation to mainstreaming transparency in independent governance and the latter in relation to revamping training and career structures.

Legislation on *health financing* can relate to any of the modes of financing health, discussed in the relevant chapter. In relation to revenue allocations for health, the Fiscal Responsibility and Debt Limitation Act 2005, stipulates the level of revenue expenditure for health and sets a target for incremental increases over the next 10 years. Revenue earmarking and public financing targets can also be part of overarching health legislation, as has previously been described. Additionally, there are two important areas for legislation relevant to increasing the base of public sources of financing for health in line with the discussion in the chapter on *Health Financing*. One relates to changes in labour laws to enhance contributions into insurance pools whereas the other involves health equity legislation in order to mandate the creation of a health equity fund. The latter is of particular importance in view of the predominance of workers in the informal sector and constraints with regard to the use of insurance as a means of pooling.

11.3.4 Personal and product liability litigation and legislation

The law of tort as administered in pre-independence India and Pakistan was based on the English common law.[380] Pakistan, being a former British colony, still follows the common law system as part of which the law of torts and damages is largely based on development of—judge made—case law. However, public litigation on this subject has not been a priority in Pakistan, unlike some other more legally developed jurisdictions following the common law system, which have achieved significant milestones in the development of this area of the law. English courts, for instance, have been regularly updating and developing the concept of the tort of negligence since 1932 while we find observations from the superior courts of Pakistan as recently as 2006 noting the need to develop this area of the law.[381] In 2006, the Supreme Court of Pakistan observed 'Our Constitution contains Chapter 1 relating to Fundamental Rights in which life of a human being is given due importance. It requires everyone to work for the welfare of the people of Pakistan but a person who is violating the law and Constitution works against the welfare of the people that is why it is high time to promote the law of tort so that the people must understand that we cannot live as a Nation without performing our duties within the framework of law.'[382]

Although the frequency of court claims in tort has remained low and the development of case law has been slow, it has not been completely ignored. The Supreme Court of Pakistan, for example, has set out the standard of care to be provided by medical professionals, 'to be one that patients should be shown a fair, reasonable, and competent degree of skill although there is no need to show that the highest degree of skill was used.'[383] There has also been some legislation in the broader context of consumer protection in Pakistan, which specifically seeks to protect consumers of goods as well as services—specifically including medical services. Although it appears that the machinery for implementation of the Islamabad Consumers Protection Act 1995 may not have been effectively put into place, the more recently promulgated law in the Punjab—the Punjab Consumer Protection Act 2005—has been implemented more faithfully with establishment of separate Consumer Courts in the province. The slow pace of development of the law of tort in Pakistan and recourse to litigation to enforce product and professional liability claims is also linked—at least in part—to the absence of comprehensive liability insurance by manufacturers and professionals, which is the norm in more legally developed jurisdictions where such litigation is more pervasive. The lack of awareness of the remedies available under the existing law of tort to consumers of goods and services is another reason for the relatively small number of claims. The Supreme Court of Pakistan has itself noted the need for cultivating awareness of these rights, particularly the law of tort.[384] An increase in the frequency of such claims can reasonably be expected to have a direct impact on service delivery and health outcomes.

Strengthening the tort system becomes critically important in Pakistan's environment where breaches of ethics in medical care are widely established. In strengthening personal and product liability litigation, the prime objective should be to improve quality of patient safety practices. An unnecessary intimidating liability environment should not be created while doing so.

In summary, legislation of relevance to health is not fully developed in Pakistan. The envisaged Reform Agenda necessitates promulgation of laws, which can enable the state to achieve its responsibility of delivering health, universally. To achieve this objective, health legislation must proceed in tandem with policy and institutional reform in the health sector. However, it must be appreciated that the most critical challenge in the health sector is not the absence of laws but poor implementation of existing laws. This is reflective of overarching socio-political issues in the country, which have a strong bearing on the state's ability to deliver any service and are amenable to reform at a much more overarching level—one that is beyond the scope of healthcare.

CHAPTER 12

The Reform Agenda

The purpose of this chapter is to consolidate the multidimensional aspects of reform outlined in different health systems domains in various sections of this publication into a unifying framework, which enables illustration of the mutually reinforcing nature of interventions proposed in various streams. The chapter consolidates the *Reform Agenda* and sets forth actionable steps, which can be implemented in a phased manner.

Before embarking on a discussion specific to these aspects of health reform, it must be recognized that health is an inter-sectoral responsibility and that isolated changes within the healthcare system can only have a limited impact. Improvements in social and general living conditions and overall state functioning can have a more profound impact on health—the former impacts health status directly whereas the latter is critical to ensuring the success of reform within the health sector. Pakistan is challenged on both these accounts. In addition, there are many other impediments to implementing a reform process in Pakistan's environment. These can be summarized as follows.

First is the country's political, law and order, and geostrategic situation, which has overwhelmed the state apparatus and has crowded out the space for structural changes relevant to the social sectors. Unfortunately, the importance of the need to reform social sector systems of the state is not fully appreciated as being critical to fighting the current divides and conflicts.

The second impediment is the current *macroeconomic downturn*, which has barely been rescued by the International Monetary Fund.[385] Pakistan was not hit hard by the global financial downturn as were many countries of South East Asia, because of the lack of integration of its financial markets with the global financial system. However, the cumulative effect of many other factors—in particular, the domino effect of many ongoing domestic crises and the global commodity crisis—has been negative on our economy. Although donors have made an exception by signalling intent to increase rather than decrease aid within this fiscally constrained milieu, however, reliance on development assistance to finance much of the social sector outlays in the 2009/10 budget makes it a highly unsustainable approach, particularly when there are no guarantees that donor pledges will be realized. Therefore, despite the expansionary fiscal policy articulated in the budget, fiscal space constraints are expected to prevail. Limited fiscal space is one of the key impediments to implementation of the envisaged *Reform Agenda*, given that its directions call for enhancing financing for health, building the capacity of state agencies, and increasing investments in human resource—all of which will require some level of scaling up of resources.

Thirdly, the most important impediment to reform is the country's public sector institutional culture, which remains focused on short-term goals as opposed to evidence-based long-term enduring actions with potential to bring sustainable change. Governance in the country is additionally weak and technical capacity to cascade multidimensional changes in a coordinated fashion, into policies, laws, and institutional arrangements is limited. The chapter on the *History of Health Reform* has outlined a plethora of initiatives under various health system domains, implemented by various governments and development agencies, over time—not one has lent impetus to transformational change that could sustainably improve healthcare delivery in the country. The pervasive culture of graft and collusion and the tendency to use decision-making prerogatives for patronage and personal gains are an impediment to institutionalization of a reform process, which necessitates a firm grounding of decisions in evidence and a long-term commitment to ensuring that decisions are implemented in their true spirit.

In the fourth place, the process of reform also faces challenges in view of technical vis-à-vis political considerations, tussles, and trade-offs, which underpin the directions of reform. Often, there is a need to reconcile equity and efficiency; harmonize the evidence-based public good character of interventions with results oriented imperatives and priorities; tackle sustainability and political expediency trade-offs; balance desirable outcome orientation with visible outputs, which usually characterize political agendas; view costs of lifesaving technologies in view of current resource constrains, and balance resource allocations for existing pressing needs with emerging challenges. The nature of some of the resulting trade-offs is opposed to long-term remedial actions.

Lastly, there appears to be no institutional memory or commitment to build on work in the pipeline and consolidate efforts underway. Successive governments tend to adopt options while subsequent governments disregard them. Information summarized in the chapter on the *History of Health Reform*, triangulated with the analysis summarized in Part II of this book, indicates that it has almost become a given for those in political roles to prioritize planning based on what is politically expedient, and for those in administrative roles not to confront them because of the fear of undue accountability or complacency. The analysis indicates that the institutional environment is, therefore, increasingly being focused on short-term objectives as a norm.

These limitations notwithstanding, it must be recognized that it has now become an imperative to reform health systems allied mechanisms of social service delivery. Pakistan's unique geostrategic challenges are calling for measures to target benefits, as this can be the only means of protecting a deeply divided society from exploitation. However, as opposed to this, the capacity to target social services has been deeply eroded. These systemic flaws underscore the need to address these challenges, no matter what the cost and how difficult the course.

12.1 The Reform Agenda: Priority areas

The *Reform Agenda* outlined in this publication has a multidimensional character (Table 14). It recognizes that reform within the healthcare sector is a profoundly political process and that reform as a public policy agenda should be tailored to the local context with respect to economic realties, political circumstances, and administrative capacities of local institutions. It further acknowledges that reform within the health sector is critically dependent on the effectiveness of overall governance and macroeconomic and political stability. It places emphasis on structural reform of the state and demonstrates the linkages of systemic reform of governance and social sector reform with reform in the health sector. Within this framework, it calls for introduction of a set of interdependent and mutually supporting interventions within the healthcare sector

Table 14. The Reform Agenda—a snapshot

Governance
Promote transparency in governance within the state system through reform of public and civil service and financial management
Institutionally reform stewardship agencies in order to enhance capacities; clear demarcation of normative, regulatory, and implementation roles; adequate resourcing at all levels and greater inter-sectoral collaboration, particularly with reference to the population-health institutional disconnect
Financing
Broaden the base of public sources of financing; increase revenues to finance basic services as a public good; improve fund utilization and reduce opportunities for corruption
Provide comprehensive coverage to the informally employed by broadening the base of social protection for health and ensuring transparency in targeting
Maximize pooling for the formally employed by expanding existing pooling platforms and mandating and incentivizing employers to cover employees
Strategically use purchasing as a tool to maximize effectiveness in service delivery
Channel predictable development assistance to help strengthen systems with a view to ultimately transition away from such support; promote debt forgiveness as a tool to free up resources for health and other social sectors
Service delivery
Expand the focus of PHC through a three-pronged approach—restructuring management of existing FLCFs, broadening the first point of contact by harnessing the outreach of private providers, and expanding the set of services to MDG+
Decentralize management and governance of public hospitals and mainstream private sector management principles to improve quality, albeit while using public sector resources to support equity objectives
Strategically use behaviour change communication, social marketing, and reform of payment systems to support restructuring of PHC and hospitals
Health related human resource
Address critical shortfalls in tandem with retention regulation
Focus on merit based hiring, appropriate placements, creating an enabling milieu, and institutionalizing accountability to reform human resource management
Review and update education, training, and capacity-building; institutionalize professional self-development and depoliticize educational institutions
Health information systems
Strengthen capacity to generate and utilize evidence for decision-making

Continued...

Table 14. Continued...

Leverage key opportunities—integrate epidemic surveillance activities, build population and registry-based surveillance, bridge gaps in the cause-of-death system, consolidate existing survey capacity, address key gaps of the HMIS, institutionalize health policy and systems research, and support research in academic settings
Strengthen capacity of the system to comply with international health regulations
Medicines, products, and related technologies
Update the law and policy in view of contemporary considerations
Reform instruments of governance in order to limit space for maneuverability and collusion in quality and price regulation by clearly separating functions of policy-making, regulation, and implementation
Make strategic use of distribution chain security, differential pricing, and flexibilities under the TRIPS Agreement
Promote ethical conduct in marketing and increase responsiveness to manufacturing impediments
Technology
Strategically use technology in health information systems to optimize time and costs, increase connectivity, and reduce errors
Leverage technology to revolutionize learning, continuing medical education, and information dissemination
Use technology to promote efficiency in the delivery of services; reduce medical costs and errors and minimize leakages and pilferages from the system

in order to institutionalize change at the structural, programmatic, institutional, and legislative levels.

The *Reform Agenda* articulates five *priory areas.* First and foremost, it underscores the need for a multi-stakeholder 'sign-up' to a *Reform Agenda.* An inclusive and participatory process should garner consensus of multipartisan stakeholders, development partners, the establishment, and the civil society on a roadmap for reform and structure multi-stakeholder oversight of the process of its implementation to ensure that reform outlives administrations and is not held hostage to vested interest. The government has recently adopted the 'All Parties Conference' approach to consensus building with reference to the current conflict in the Northern Areas of the country.[386] This style of consensus building can be broadened to include other stakeholders and the civil society to build a consensus on the reform agenda. This is a critical prerequisite to any substantive action with reference to reform.

The second priority is to address broader constraints within the remit of the political economy and inequities of power, money, and resources, which are one of the strongest determinants of health status achievement.[387] Debt limitation, fiscal responsibility, and measures to broaden the tax base are necessary in order to create the needed fiscal space for the health sector. Macroeconomic reform is critical for pro-poor macroeconomic growth and bridging broader social inequities whereas measures to promote transparency in overall governance through reform of public and civil service and financial management can deeply impact health systems performance.

Thirdly, increasing the base of public sources of financing for health is deemed critical. Measures can include incremental increases in revenues earmarked for health to support essential services, broadening the base of social protection for the informally employed sector, and maximizing pooling through insurance for the formally employed sector. Increase in funding, coupled with strategic approaches to public service delivery management reengineering, can help in achieving two end points. On the one hand, with appropriate incentives and accountability arrangements, workforce can be retained in the public sector, whereas on the other hand, with the help of transparency in management, procurement, and supply chains, availability of essential medicines and supplies can be enhanced and infrastructure improved. Options can be developed for better management of public facilities, incentivization of directly managed services and granting of greater operational autonomy with appropriate oversight or contracting out, albeit with appropriate safeguards.

In the fourth place, market harnessing regulatory approaches have been flagged as a priority. These can enable both harnessing the outreach of non-state providers in order to broaden the first point of contact in Primary Health Care as well as enable purchase of services in order to achieve equity in the delivery of care, more broadly. These changes in service delivery and financing arrangements necessitate institutional reform of state agencies mandated in a health role in order to enhance their normative and oversight capacity to oversee provision of services, ideally with institutional separation of policy-making, implementation and regulatory functions.

Lastly, broader directions for reforming public and market service delivery arrangements should be complemented with additional measures. Notable amongst these are the strategic use of technology. In the case of medicines and products, technology can secure the distribution chain and assist with making procurements transparent and efficient. In health information systems, technology can optimize time and increase connectivity, whereas in the space of training and education, technology can revolutionize training, continuing medial education and information dissemination.

12.2 The Reform Agenda: Phasing implementation

The five priority areas of the *Reform Agenda* articulated in this publication can be implemented in a *phased approach* as is being outlined in Table 15. It must be recognized, however, that there can be significant overlap between these phases and that the delineation proposed herein is part of an effort to demonstrate how complex interrelated measures can be sequenced, and taken one at a time, while being integral to a holistic process.

Step 1 should focus on two measures—*developing a national consensus on the Reform Agenda* and *increasing public financing for health*. The need for consensus over a reform agenda and an oversight mechanism to ensure that the consensus driven agenda is implemented in its true spirit can be the single most important factor in determining the success of reform, as already outlined. By garnering consensus over the directions for an envisaged reform, safeguards can be built against detracking and retracking, which has been characteristic of the institutional history of the process of reform, as has been explained in the chapter on the *History of Health Reform in Pakistan*. More importantly, the consensus building effort can impact the directions for reform within the remit of governance and social sector systems, more broadly, which as has been explained earlier, deeply impact health status and performance of the health system. Key transparency promoting measures—both within as well as outside of the health sector—need to be an inherent part of this approach and can supplement other transparency promoting measures, specific to the health sector in Step III.

Measures to enhance public financing for health should also be initialized in Step I. This can signal support for the process and ensure a reasonable fiscal basis for the planned changes. Measures should

Table 15. Phase-wise implementation of the Reform Agenda

STEP I
Developing a national consensus on the reform agenda
Increasing public financing for health
Incremental increase in the health budget and allocations for health in the social protection pool
Regulatory interventions in the labour market
STEP II
Bracing the health information system
Designation and appropriate resourcing of a health information apex arrangement
Initiation of work to integrate epidemic surveillance activities; address key weaknesses of death surveillance; expand DHIS; consolidate survey capacity and establish a mechanism for periodic assessment of health systems performance
Pulling a thread through existing evidence
Analysis of existing evidence in key health systems domains to guide changes in specific areas—Primary Health Care and hospital restructuring arrangements; initiatives that have experimented with strategic purchasing, social and community health insurance, and other forms of pooling to fund exemptions and systems innovations in health and related areas
STEP III
Strengthening institutions
Strengthening capacity and reconfiguring role of stewardship agencies
Demarcating and/or establishing well-resourced implementing and regulatory agencies
Achieving clarity in roles, responsibilities, and prerogatives at the three levels of government
Creation of an effective inter-sectoral collaborating mechanism
Mainstreaming population planning into essential health services
Honing norms
Updating the Drug Policy; formulating a policy on human resource and information
Updating the Drug Act and public health legislation
Enacting legislation/standards to establish norms of public-private relationships, equity in financing, marketing and promotion, and strengthening of personal and product liability litigation
Establishing key regulations outside of the health sector—incentivizing employers and private insurance agencies; black market curbs, device regulation, and others as appropriate
Mainstreaming technology
Making investments in technology to eliminate pilferages, improve efficiency and connectivity, control costs, reduce errors, and facilitate implementation of new services
STEP IV Prototyping alternative service delivery and financing mechanisms
STEP IV Upscaling

include a plan for incremental increases in revenues earmarked for health directly as well as through the social protection pool. In addition, regulatory interventions in the labour market can be a good starting point to secure health coverage for a higher number of individuals.

Step II should centre on *bracing the health information system* and *pulling a thread through existing evidence.* As part of the former, designation and appropriate resourcing and mandating of a health information apex arrangement and initiation of work to bridge gaps in existing health information channels are important. The latter should focus on integrating epidemic surveillance activities, addressing key weaknesses of death surveillance, expanding the scope of the District Health Information System with web-based connectivity, consolidating survey capacity and establishing a mechanism for periodic assessment of health systems performance and its institutionalization. Timely initiation of these steps should be a priority. However, since these measures would take time to fully implement and institutionalize, they should not deter the initiation of other steps.

Step II should also pull a thread through existing evidence in key health systems domains to guide changes in specific areas. These areas include Primary Health Care and hospital restructuring arrangements, initiatives that have experimented with strategic purchasing, social and community health insurance, and other forms of pooling to fund exemptions and systems innovations in health and related areas.

Step III is envisioned as encompassing three important elements—*strengthening institutional capacity; honing norms and standards,* and *mainstreaming the use of technology in the health system.* Institutional capacity strengthening has many dimensions in it own right, as has been outlined in Table 14. Appropriate resources and structural changes are a prerequisite for each. In order to sustainably improve health systems performance, reconfiguration of the role of stewardship agencies and augmentation of their normative and oversight role is an imperative. In tandem, regulatory and implementing agencies should be demarcated as autonomous entities and should be adequately resourced to perform clearly mandated roles. While doing so, the federal, provincial, and district roles and responsibilities need to be clearly demarcated and effective inter-sectoral coordinating mechanisms need to be established. The opportunity to structure institutional arrangements should be capitalized to introduce family planning as part of essential services in healthcare delivery.

Step III should also focus on honing norms and standards. Many areas such as the National Drug Policy, the Drug Act 1976, and public health legislation relevant to many areas need to be updated whereas new statutes/standards need to be established in key financing, service delivery, marketing and promotion, and human resource-related areas. Regulations, policies and norms outside of the health sector, particularly in case of the labour and drug market, are also needed as part of the envisaged reform process and can be structured during this phase. Mainstreaming technology is the third major element of Step III. Technology should be used on a priority basis to plug leakages and pilferages from the system and promote overall transparency in governance. Other uses of technology, which can enable gains in efficiency, cost control, reduction in error, facilitation of new services and improvements in connectivity should also be promoted and investments in these areas supported.

Step IV should be dedicated to *implementing appropriate changes in existing pilots and prototyping in key settings to develop best practice models*. Prototypes should centre on the following areas: (a) management restructuring of FLCFs by introducing elements of competition as an incentive for improving performance and quality, both in contracting out arrangements to non-state entities as well as intra-organizational contracting in directly managed services; (b) harnessing the outreach of private providers to deliver essential services through market harnessing regulatory arrangements. In both (a) and (b) a predefined package of essential services, inclusive of family planning, should be used as a service delivery target; (c) management reform of public hospitals centred on effective use of private sector management principles, albeit with equity and quality in service delivery as its key principles. The idea in all of the above is to strengthen the oversight role of stewardship agencies and build capacity within the districts to choose appropriate restructuring arrangements based on locally suited options; (d) broadening the base of the ESSI to include a wider segment of the population; (e) effective targeting mechanisms for waivers in hospitals; (f) models for strategic purchasing from state and non-state entities, and (g) human resource arrangements that can balance an enabling milieu with accountability. **Step V** should facilitate up-scaling of prototypes.

Implementation of the multidimensional nature of reform envisaged by these directions necessitates political will, perseverance, consistency of policy directions over time, and the resolve and capacity to cascade multidimensional changes into policies, laws, and institutional arrangements. Limited capacity, short-term outlook of governments, and lack of transparency in governance create impediments to institutionalization of these changes. The importance of these impediments to systemic reform must be appreciated in aiming for economic stability for the country, welfare of its people, and a positive proactive role of Pakistan in a globalized world.

References

1. Ravishankar N, Gubbins P, Cooley RJ, Leach-Kemon K, Michaud CM, Jamison DT, et al. Financing of global health: tracking development assistance for health from 1990-2007. *Lancet* 2009;373:2113-24.

2. Schellenberg D. In: Specter M. What money can buy. *The New Yorker* 2005; October 24: 57-71. http://www.michaelspecter.com/ny/2005/2005/1024gates.html. (accessed Oct. 02, 09).

3. Murray CJL, Frenk J. A framework for assessing the performance of health systems. *Bull World Health Organ* 2000;78:717-31.

4. Frenk J. Institutions in context: strengthening health systems as the next step for global progress. *PLoS Medicine*, (Forthcoming).

5. United Nations. The Millennium Development Goals Report, 2006. New York, USA: United Nations, 2006. http://mdgs.un.org/unsd/mdg/Resources/Static/Products/Progress2006/MDGReport2006.pdf (accessed April 07, 09).

6. World Health Organization Maximizing Positive Synergies Collaborative Group. Samb B, Evans T, Dybul M, Atun R, Moatti JP, Nishtar S, Wright A, Celletti F, Hsu J, Kim JY, Brugha R, Russell A, Etienne C. An assessment of interactions between global health initiatives and country health systems. *Lancet* 2009;373(9681):2137-69.

7. Nishtar S. Mixed Health Systems Syndrome. *Bull World Health Organ* 2009 (Forthcoming).

8. World Health Organization. WHO's framework for Action: Everybody's Business—Strengthening health systems to improve health outcomes. Geneva, Switzerland: WHO, 2007. http://www.searo.who.int/LinkFiles/Health_Systems_EverybodyBusinessHSS.pdf (accessed April 07, 09).

9. Memorandum of Understanding on developing the National Health Policy. Ministry of Health, Government of Pakistan; World Health Organization, Heartfile and Pakistan's Health Policy Forum: Islamabad, 2007. http://heartfile.org/ (accessed Oct. 19, 07).

10. Biehl J, Petryna A, Gertner A, Amon JJ, Picon PD. Judicialisation of the right to health in Brazil. *Lancet* 2009;373(9682):2182-4.

11. Byrne I. Enforcing the right to health: innovative lessons from domestic courts. In: Clapham A, Robinson M, Mahon C, Jerbi S, editors. Realizing the right to health. Zurich, Switzerland: Rüffer & Rub; 2009, pp. 525-38.

12. 11th session of the United Nations Human Rights Council. Preventable maternal mortality and morbidity and human rights. Geneva, 2–19 June 2009. http://www2.ohchr.org/english/bodies/hrcouncil/11session/ (accessed July 10, 09).

13. United Nations General Assembly. Convention on the Rights of the Child, 1989. Document A/RES/44/25. http://www.cirp.org/library/ethics/UN-convention/ (accessed March 26, 08).

14. United Nations General Assembly. The Convention on the Elimination of All Forms of Discrimination against Women, 1979. http://www.un.org/womenwatch/daw/cedaw/ (accessed March 26, 08).

15. Declaration of Alma Ata. International Conference on Primary Health Care; 1978 Sep. 6-12; Alma Ata, USSR; 1978. http://www.euro.who.int/AboutWHO/Policy/20010827_1 (accessed March 26, 08).

16. UNFPA: United Nation Population fund. Programme of Action of the International Conference on Population and Development; Cairo; 1994. http://www.unfpa.org/icpd/summary.htm (accessed March 26, 08).

17. The United Nations Fourth World Conference on Women. Platform for Action; Beijing; 1995. http://www.iwhc.org/global/un/unhistory/fwcw.cfm (accessed March 26, 08).

18. Miss Shehla Zia and others v. WAPDA [PLD 1994 Supreme Court 693].

19. Syed Mansoor Ali Shah v. Government of Punjab [2007 C. L. D.533].

20. Nishtar S. Judicialisation of rights. The News International 2009 July 25; sect. comment:6. http://www.thenews.com.pk/editorial_detail.asp?id=189757 (accessed Sep. 25, 09).

21. Clapham A, Robinson M, Mahon C, Jerbi S, editors. Realizing the Right to health. Switzerland: Rüffer & Rub; 2009.

22. Cassels A. Health Sector Reform: Key issues in less developed countries. *J Int Dev* 1995;7(3): 329-47.

23. Berman P. Health sector reform: making health development sustainable. *Health Policy* 1995;32(1):13-28.

24. Barack Obama and Joe Biden's plan to lower health care costs and ensure affordable, accessible health coverage for all. http://www.barackobama.com/pdf/issues/HealthCareFullPlan.pdf (accessed March 26, 09).

25. Loevinsohn B, Harding A. Buying results? Contracting for health service delivery in developing countries. *Lancet* 2005;366(9486):676-81.

26. Palmer N. The use of private sector contracts for primary health care: theory, evidence, and lessons for low-income and middle-income countries. *Bull World Health Organ* 2000;78(6):821-9.

27. Mills A. To contract or not to contract? Issues for low and middle-income countries. *Health Policy Plan* 1998;13(1):32-40.

28. White J. Protecting Medicare: the best defence is a good offence. *J Health Polit Policy Law* 2007;32(2):221-46.

29. Scrivens E. The role of regulation and governance. *J R Soc Health* 2007;127(2):72-7.

30. Whitehead M, Dahlgren G, Evans T. Equity and health sector reforms: can low-income countries escape the medical poverty trap? *Lancet* 2001;358(9284):833-6.

31. Waitzkin H, Jasso-Aguilar R, Iriart C. Privatization of health services in less developed countries: an empirical response to the proposals of the World Bank and Wharton School. *Int J Health Serv* 2007;37(2):205-27.

32. Wagstaff A. Health systems in East Asia: what can developing countries learn from Japan and the Asian Tigers? *Health Econ* 2007;16(5):441-56.

33. De Vos P, De Ceukelaire W, Van der Stuyft P. Columbia and Cuba, contrasting models in Latin America's health sector reform. *Trop Med Int Health* 2006;11(10):1604-12.

34. Lagomarsino G, de Ferranti D, Pablos-Mendez A, Nachuk S, Nishtar S, Wibulpolprasert S. Public stewardship of Mixed Health Systems. *Lancet* 2009 Aug 11. [Epub ahead of print].

35. Kunhikannan TP, Aravindan KP. Changes in the health status of Kerala 1987-1997. Discussion paper No 20. Thiruvananthapuram: Kerala research programme on local level development, Centre for development studies; 2000. http://www.krpcds.org/kunhikannan.pdf (accessed Aug. 08, 08).

36. Horwitz A. Comparative public health: Costa Rica, Cuba and Chile. Washington DC, USA: World Health Organization, 1986. http://www.unu.edu/unupress/food/8f093e/8F093E04.htm (accessed Aug. 08, 08).

37. De Vos P. "No one left abandoned": Cuba's national health system since the 1959 revolution. *Int J Health Serv* 2005;35(1):189-207.

38. The World Bank. Success in addressing priorities, priorities in health. Washington D.C, USA: The World Bank, 2006. http://files.dcp2.org/pdf/PIH/PIH.pdf (accessed Dec. 11, 08).

39. Fitzner KA, Coughlin S, Tomori C, Bennett CL. Health care in Hong Kong and Mainland China: one country, two systems? *Health Policy* 2000;53(3):147-55.

40. Damrongplasit K, Melnick AG. Early results from Thailand's 30 Baht health reform: Something to smile about. *Health Aff (Millwood)*. 2009 May-Jun;28(3):w457-66. Epub. 2009 March 31.

41. Prince Mahidol Award Foundation. Three decades of primary health care: reviewing the past and defining the future. Proceedings of the Prince Mahidol Award Conference: 2008 Jan 30-Feb 01; Bangkok, Thailand.

42. Fernald LCH, Gertler PJ, Neufeld LM. Role of conditional cash transfer programs for child health, growth and development: an analysis of Mexico's Oportunidades. *Lancet* 2008;371:828-37.

43. De Savigny D, Kasale H, Mbuya C, Reid G. Fixing health systems, 2nd ed. Ottawa, Canada: International Development Research Centre, 2008. http://www.idrc.ca/openebooks/411-6/ (accessed Dec. 31, 08).

44. Atun RA. Privatization as decentralization strategy. In: Saltman R, Bankauskaite V, Vrangbaek K, editors. Decentralization in health care: strategies and outcomes. Berkshire and New York: Open University Press; 2007.

45. Boerma W, Dubois C. Mapping primary care across Europe. In: Saltman R, Rico A, Boerma W, editors. Primary care in the driver's seat? Organizational reform in European primary care. Berkshire and New York: Open University Press, 2006.

46. Ibid., ref. no. 15.

47. Walsh J, Werner K. Selective Primary Health Care, an interim strategy for disease control in the developing countries. *NEJM* 1979;301:967-74.

48. Nishtar S. Public Private partnerships in health – a global call to action. In: Commonwealth health ministers book. London, United Kingdom: 2007. http://heartfile.org/pdf/ppp_commonwealth.pdf. (accessed Dec. 12, 08).

49. Commission of the European communities. From Monterrey to the European Consensus on Development: honouring our commitments. Brussels, 2007. http://register.consilium.europa.eu/pdf/en/07/st08/st08340.en07.pdf (accessed Dec. 12, 08).

50. Ibid., ref. no. 5.

51. National Programme for Prevention and Control of Hepatitis, Ministry of Health, Pakistan. http://www.health.gov.pk/(accessed May 26, 09).

52. National Programme for the Prevention and Control of Blindness. Ministry of Health, Pakistan. http://www.health.gov.pk/(accessed May 26, 09).

53. Nishtar S. National Action Plan for Prevention and Control of Non-Communicable Diseases and Health Promotion in Pakistan. Islamabad, Pakistan: Heartfile, Ministry of Health, Government of Pakistan and World Health Organization; 2004. http://heartfile.org/pdf/NAPmain.pdf (accessed April 07, 09).

54. The United States President's Emergency Plan for AIDS Relief. http://www.pepfar.gov/countries/index.htm (accessed May 25, 09).

55. World Health Organization. The World Health Report 2000: Health systems—improving performance. Geneva, Switzerland: WHO, 2000. http://www.who.int/whr/2000/en/ (accessed July 17, 08).

56. Chen L, Evans T, Anand S, Boufford JI, Brown H, Chowdhury M, et al. Human resources for health: overcoming the crisis. *Lancet* 2004;364(9449):1984-90.

57. World Health Organization. The Montreux Challenge: Making health systems work. Glion-sur-Montreux, Switzerland: WHO, 2005.

58. Chan M. Opening remarks at the high-level consultation. Scaling up research and learning for better health: 02 June 2008; Divonne Les Bains, France. http://www.who.int/dg/speeches/2008/20080602b/en/ (accessed July 01, 08).

59. World Health Organization. Maximizing Positive Synergies Between Health Systems and Global Health Initiatives. Geneva, Switzerland: Health Systems and Services, WHO, 2008. htttp://www.who.int/healthsystems/GHIsynergies/en/ (accessed Sep. 22, 08).

60. Bamako Call to Action. http://unesdoc.unesco.org/images/0017/001777/177791m.pdf (accessed Nov. 26, 08).

61. World Health Organization. World Health Report 2008: Primary Health Care—Now More Than Ever. Geneva, Switzerland: WHO, 2008. http://www.who.int/whr/2008/whr08_en.pdf (accessed March 13, 09).

62. Commission on Social Determinants of Health. Closing the gap in a generation: health equity through action on the social determinants of health. Geneva, Switzerland: WHO, 2008. / http://whqlibdoc.who.int/publications/2008/9789241563703_eng.pdf (accessed Nov. 25, 08).

63. World Health Organization. The Tallinn Charter: health systems for health and wealth. Proceedings of WHO European ministerial conference on health systems: 2008 June 25-7; Tallinn, Estonia. 2008. http://www.euro.who.int/document/E91438.pdf (accessed May 20, 09).

64. World Health Organization. Ouagadougou Declaration on Primary Health Care and health systems in Africa: achieving better health for Africa in the new millennium: Burkina Faso, 28-30 April 2008. http://www.afro.who.int/phc_hs_2008/documents/En/Ouagadougou%20 declaration%20version%20Eng.pdf (accessed May 20, 09).

65. Horton R. Venice statement: global health initiatives and health systems. *Lancet* 2009;374(9683):10-12.

66. Atun R, Dybul M, Evans T, Kim JY, Moatti JP, Nishtar S, Russell A. Venice Statement on global health initiatives and health systems. *Lancet* 2009;374(9692):783-4.

67. Global Alliance for Vaccines and Immunization. Health Systems Strengthening. http://www.gavialliance.org/support/what/hss/index.php (accessed June 27, 08).

68. Investing in our future. The Global Fund to Fight AIDS, Tuberculosis and Malaria; National Strategy Application. http://www.theglobalfund.org/en/ (accessed June 27, 08).

69. World Health Organization. Health Metrics Network. http://www.who.int/healthmetrics/ (accessed June 27, 08).

70. World Health Organization. Global Workforce Alliance. http://www.ghwa.org/ (accessed June 27, 08).

71. International Health Partnership. http://www.internationalhealthpartnership.net/index.html (accessed April 07, 09).

72. Paris Declaration on Aid effectiveness. http://www.oecd.org/dataoecd/11/41/34428351.pdf/ (accessed June 27, 08).

73. Accra Agenda for Action. http://siteresources.worldbank.org/ACCRAEXT/Resources/4700790-1217425866038/AAA-4-SEPTEMBER-FINAL-16h00.pdf (accessed Sep. 23, 08).

74. The Rockefeller Foundation, Results for Development and the International Health Policy Programme, Thailand. Role of the private sector in health systems. http://www.rockfound.org/library/020108private_sector_health.pdf/ (accessed June 27, 08).

75. Doris Duke Charitable Foundation. Operations Research in AIDS Care and Treatment in Africa Programme. http://www.ddcf.org/page.asp?pageId=486 (accessed Oct. 09, 08).

76. Reich MR, Takemi K. G8 and strengthening of health systems: follow-up to the Toyako summit. *Lancet* 2009;373(9662):508-15.

77. G 8 Health Experts Group. Toyako Framework for Action on Global Health. Toyako, Japan: Ministry of Foreign Affairs of Japan, 2008. http://www.mofa.go.jp/policy/economy/summit/2008/doc/pdf/0708_09_en.pdf (accessed April 07, 08).

78. Nishtar S. The Gateway Paper: Health Systems in Pakistan—a Way Forward. Islamabad, Pakistan: Heartfile, 2006. http://heartfile.org/pdf/phpf-GWP.pdf (accessed April 07, 09).

79. Ibid., ref. no. 9.

80. Finance Division, Government of Pakistan. Chapter 9 - Pillar VI: Human development for the 21st century. In: Poverty Reduction Strategy Paper-II. Islamabad, Pakistan: Government of Pakistan; 2009. p. 173. http://www.finance.gov.pk/admin/images/poverty/PRSP-II.pdf (accessed May 25, 09).

81. Nishtar S. Pablos-Mendez A. The Global Financial downturn—imperatives for the health sector. *Lancet* 2009;373:124.

82. White House White Paper on U.S. policy to Afghanistan and Pakistan. http://thecable.foreignpolicy.com/posts/2009/03/27/white_house_white_paper_on_us_policy_to_afghanistan_and_pakistan (accessed April 06, 09).

83. Ibid., ref. no. 67.

84. Ministry of Health, Government of Pakistan. Zero draft, National Health Policy 2009: Stepping Towards Better Health. http://www.healthnwfp.gov.pk/downloads/draft%20health%20policy.pdf (accessed May 20, 09).

85. National Commission for Government Reforms. Reforms on reforming the government in Pakistan. Islamabad, Pakistan: Prime Minister's secretariat, Government of Pakistan, 2008. http://www.ncgr.gov.pk/ (accessed June 10, 08).

86. Gtz—partner for future, worldwide. http://www.gtz.de/en/weltweit/europa-kaukasus-zentralasien/18669.htm (accessed March 28, 08).

87. Asian Development Bank. Technical assistance to Pakistan for health sector reform in North-West Frontier Province. Asian Development Bank, 2000. http://www.adb.org/Documents/TARs/PAK/R34-00.pdf (accessed July 09, 08).

88. Asian Development Bank. Technical Assistance Completion Report: January 2001–Health sector reform in the North-West Frontier Province. Asian Development Bank, 2000. htttp://www.adb.org/Documents/TACRs/PAK/tacr_pak_3386.pdf (accessed July 09, 08).

89. The World Bank. World Bank provides US $451 million to support Pakistan's development programme. Pakistan Press release June 08, 2007. http://www.worldbank.org.pk (accessed Aug. 01, 08).

90. The World Bank. World Bank approves $ 90 million to support second phase of reforms in North-West Frontier Province. Pakistan; Press release Jun 22, 2004. http://www.worldbank.org.pk (accessed Aug. 01, 08).

91. Government of Punjab. Poverty Focused Investment Strategy for Punjab, Pakistan. http://www.punjab-prmp.gov.pk/pfis/Documents/PFIS.Main.Report.Final.Version(Volume-I).pdf (accessed March 28, 08).

92. Punjab Resource Management Programme. Health Sector Reform Framework. Lahore, Pakistan: Planning and Development department, Government of Punjab, 2006. http://202.83.162.250/prmp-documents/publications/HealthSectorReformFramework.pdf (accessed March 28, 08).

93. Punjab Devolved Social Services Programme. http://www.pdssp.gop.pk/ (accessed March 28, 08).

94. Punjab Resource Management Programme. http://www.punjab-prmp.gov.pk/ (accessed March 28, 08).

95. Punjab Resource Management Programme, Punjab Health Department. Consultative process for prioritization of health sector reforms interventions in Punjab. Pakistan: Government of Punjab and Asian Development Bank, 2008.

96. Government of India. Health Survey and Development Committee Report. Vol. 1-4. New Delhi, India: Ministry of Health, Government of India; 1946.

97. Ibid., ref. no. 15.

98. Planning Commission. Vision 2030. Islamabad, Pakistan. Planning Commission, Government of Pakistan, 2007. http://www.202.83.167.93/pcportal/vision2030.htm (accessed May 07, 08).

99. The World Bank. Family Health Project (02). Balochistan and Punjab Department of health, Government of Pakistan: The World Bank, 1999. http://web.worldbank.org/external/projects/main?Projectid=P010414&Type=Implementation&theSitePK=40941&pagePK=64330676&menuPK=64282137&piPK=64302789 (accessed March 28, 08).

100. The World Bank. Implementation Completion Report (TF-20383; TF-21206; TF-20716; TF-21746; IDA-30500) Second Social Action Program Project. Washington, DC: The World Bank, 2003.

101. Sofia S. Analysis of the experience of government partnerships with non-governmental organizations, Multi-donor Support Unit for SAP: The World Bank, 2002.

102. United Nations Development Programme Pakistan. Accelerating the pace of development—a case study of the Lodhran pilot project. Local initiative facility for urban environment: Islamabad, Pakistan, 2002.

103. Chief Minister's Programme for Primary Health Care. http://www.prsp-cmiphc.gov.pk/ (accessed March 28, 08).

104. President of Pakistan's Task Force on Primary Health Care: concept Paper. http://www.nchd.org.pk/ws/mat/publications/phc_cp.pdf (accessed April 30, 08).

105. People's Primary Health Care Initiative. Government of Pakistan. http://pphi-nwfpfata.org/index.php (accessed May 09, 09).

106. National Commission for Human Development. Strengthening and restructuring of Primary Health Care system and improving health of primary school students in eleven districts of Punjab. Islamabad, Pakistan: Department of Health, Government of Punjab; 2007.

107. Minimum Service Delivery Standards for Primary and Secondary Health Care. http://www.adb.org/Documents/RRPs/PAK/rrp-pak-32264.pdf (accessed May 08, 08).

108. The World Bank. Partnering with NGOs to strengthen management: an external evaluation of the Chief Minister's initiative on Primary Health Care in Rahim Yar Khan District, Punjab, Pakistan: 2006. http://web.worldbank.org/external/projects/main?menuPK=51521804&pagePK=51351007&piPK=64675967&theSitePK=40941&menuPK=64154159&searchMenuPK=51521783&theSitePK=40941&entityID=000310607_20061102141053&searchMenuPK=51521783&theSitePK=40941 (accessed May 08, 08).

109. Heard A, Chandio I, Memon R. Improving maternal health by scaling up contractual management of Basic Health Units in Sindh Province, Pakistan: a health systems approach. Commissioned paper for the International conference on scaling up. December 3-6, 2008. Dhaka, Bangladesh.

110. Heartfile. http://heartfile.org/ (accessed May 20, 09).

111. Sight Savers. http://www.sightsavers.org/our_work/around_the_world/asia/pakistan/default.html (accessed May 20, 09).

112. Maqbool S. Towards a vision for control of NCDs, once more! The News International 2009, May 01. http://www.thenews.com.pk/arc_news.asp?id=6(accessed Sep. 26, 09).

113. Evans T, Nishtar S, Atun R, Etienne C. Scaling up research and learning for health systems: time to act. *Lancet* 2008;372(9649):1529-31.

114. Ronis KA, Nishtar S. Community health promotion in Pakistan: a policy development perspective. *Promot Educ* 2007;14(2):98-9.

115. Planning Commission, Government of Pakistan. http://www.pakistan.gov.pk/ministries/planning and development-ministry/ (accessed May 08, 08).

116. Khushaal Pakistan Program, Local Government and Rural Development Division. http://www.pakistan.gov.pk/divisions/ContentInfo.jsp?DivID=45&cPath=618_621&ContentID=3270 (accessed June 23, 08).

117. Bhutta Z, editor. Maternal and Child Health in Pakistan: Challenges and Opportunities. Karachi, Pakistan: Oxford University Press; 2004.

118. Khan FJ, Javed Y. Delivering access to safe drinking water and adequate sanitation in Pakistan. In: PIDE—Working Papers 2007:30. Islamabad, Pakistan: Pakistan Institute of Development Economics, 2007. http://www.ideas.repec.org/p/pid/wpaper/200730.html (accessed June 23, 08).

119. The World Bank. Better management of Indus waters. Islamabad, Pakistan: The World Bank; 2006. http://www.siteresources.worldbank.org/INTPAKISTAN/Data%20and%20 Reference/20805819/Brief-Indus-Basin-Water.pdf (accessed June 23, 08).

120. Khattak FH. Economy of primary healthcare. In: Economics of health sector reforms in Pakistan. Islamabad, Pakistan: Ad Ray Printers, p. 45.

121. Abdullah MT, Shaw J. A review of the experience of hospital autonomy in Pakistan. *Int J Health Mgmt* 2007;22:45-62.

122. The World Bank. Pakistan, Punjab Pilot Hospital Autonomy Project (Learning and Innovation Loan) http://www-wds.worldbank.org/external/default/main?pagePK=64193027&piPK=64187937&theSitePK=523679&menuPK=64187510&searchMenuPK=64187283&siteName=WDS&entityID=000178830_98111703532683 (accessed March 27, 08).

123. Punjab Institute of Cardiology. http://www.pic.gop.pk/ (accessed April 07, 09).

124. Ibid., ref. no. 87.

125. Office of the Chief Executive. Efficiency and appraisal report KTH, KMC & KCD: 20 April 2000-19 April 2003. Peshawar, Pakistan: Khyber Teaching Hospital, 2003.

126. Sindh Institute of Urology and Transplantation. Pakistan. http://www.siut.org/ (accessed April 21, 08).

127. Sindh Devolved Social Services Program. Program Number: 34337; Loan Number: 2047/48. 2007, Pakistan. http://www.adb.org/Documents/Tranche-Releases/PAK/34337-PAK-PRTR.pdf (accessed April 21, 08).

128. Ahmad K. Private practice in Pakistan comes under fire. *Lancet* 2000;355:2145.

129. Ahmad K. Pakistan's province limits private practice in public hospitals. *Lancet* 2002;359(9307):685.

130. Supreme Court of Pakistan. Human rights case no. 3852 of 2005 (Ministry of Health). Islamabad, Pakistan: 2005.

131. Ministry of Health. Brief to the Prime Minister: Institutional based practice in government hospitals. Islamabad, Pakistan: Ministry of Health, Government of Pakistan, 2006.

132. Federal Bureau of Statistics, Statistics Division. 50 years of Pakistan. Islamabad, Pakistan: Government of Pakistan, 1998.

133. Makinen M, Ashir Z. Report on the workshop on 'Policy options for financing health services in Pakistan' Islamabad, Pakistan: USAID, 1992.

134. Weber A. Technical assistance to the Islamic Republic of Pakistan for preparing the social protection strategy development study. TAR:PAK 37008. Asian Development Bank, 2003.

135. Gesellshaft fur Versicherungswissenschaft und-gestaltung e.V (GVG). Social Protection Strategy development study. Final report Vol.11: Health insurance. ADB TA 4155-PAK: Social Protection Strategy, 2004.

136. Weber A. Technical assistance to the Islamic Republic of Pakistan for developing the social health insurance project. TAR: PAK 37359: Asian Development Bank, 2005.

137. Asian Development Bank. Social Protection Strategy development study: final report Vol II: Health insurance. ADB TA 4155-PAK: Social Protection Strategy, 2004.

138. Ministry of Social Welfare & Special Education. Social Protection Strategy, 2005. Government of Pakistan: Islamabad, Pakistan; 2005.

139. Annear PL, Wilkinson D, Men RC, Van Pelt M. Study of financial access to health services for the poor in Cambodia, Phase 1: Scope, Design, and data analysis. Phnom Penh: Ministry of Health, WHO, AusAID, RMIT University (Melbourne), 2006.

140. Annear PL, Bigdeli M, Ros CE, James P. Study of financial access to health services for the poor in Cambodia, Phase 2: In-depth analysis of selected case Studies. Phnom Penh: Ministry of Health, WHO, AusAID, RMIT University (Melbourne), 2007.

141. Sekhri N, Savedoff W, Thripathi S. Regulating private health insurance to serve the public interest – policy issues for developing countries. Geneva, Switzerland: Health System Financing and Evidence and Information for Policy, World Health Organization, 2005. http://www.who.int/health_financing/documents/dp_e_05_03-regulating_private_h_ins.pdf (accessed May 08, 09).

142. McGuiness E, Tounytsky V. The demand for micro insurance in Pakistan: Microfinance Opportunities. Washington: USA. 2006.

143. Nishtar S. Health Indicators of Pakistan—Gateway Paper II. Islamabad: Heartfile, Health Policy Forum, Statistics Division, Government of Pakistan, World Health Organization and Ministry of Health, Government of Pakistan; 2007. http://www.heartfile.org/pdf/GWP-II.pdf (accessed April 07, 09).

144. National Institute of Population Studies and Macro International Inc. Pakistan Demographic and Health Survey, 2006-07. Islamabad, Pakistan: National Institute of Population Studies and Macro International Inc, 2008.

145. Budget speech; Government of Pakistan. http://www.app.com.pk/en_/index2.php?option=com_content&do_pdf=1&id=38838 (accessed Sep. 14, 08).

146. Nishtar S. Pharmaceuticals—strategic considerations in health reforms in Pakistan. *J Pak Med Assoc* 2006;56(12 Suppl.4):S100-11.

147. The Network for Consumer Protection and *Lok Sujag*. Results of the survey to assess the impact of liberalization of policies on drug prices. *Drug Bulletin* 2001;10(3&4).

148. Federal Bureau of Statistics, Statistics Division. Respective Demographic Surveys for the years 1992-2003. Islamabad, Pakistan: Government of Pakistan. http://www.statpak.gov.pk/depts/fbs/statistics/pds2001/pds2001.html.(accessed July 18, 08).

149. National Health Management Information System, Ministry of Health, Pakistan. http://www.pakistan.gov.pk/divisions/ContentInfo.jsp?DivID=25&cPath=254_260&ContentID=1635 (accessed July 11, 08).

150. Pakistan Medical Research Council. http://www.pmrc.org.pk/ (accessed July 11, 08).

151. Ibid., ref. no. 143.

152. Ibid.

153. Collins CD, Omar M, Tarin E. Decentralization, healthcare and policy process in the Punjab, Pakistan in the 1990s. *Int J Health Plann Mgmt* 2002;17:123-46.

154. Project Management Team. The state of public sector Primary Health Care services, district Sheikhupura, Punjab, Pakistan. Bamako Initiative Technical Report Series. New York, USA: UNICEF, 1994.

155. The Local Government System, National Reconstruction Bureau, Government of Pakistan. http://www.nrb.gov.pk/local_government/default.aspNRB (accessed June 12, 08).

156. Nishtar S. Politics of health systems: WHO's new frontier. *Lancet* 2007;370(9591):935-6.

157. Ibid., ref. no. 55.

158. Ibid., ref. no. 8.

159. Finance Division. Pakistan Economic Survey, 2007. Islamabad, Pakistan: Ministry of Finance, Government of Pakistan, 2008. http://www.finance.gov.pk/survey/survey.htm (accessed May 30, 08).

160. Federal Bureau of Statistics. National Education Census, 2005. Islamabad, Pakistan: Government of Pakistan, 2005.

161. *A literate person has been defined as someone who can read a newspaper and write a simple letter in any language.*

162. Population Census Organization, Statistics Division. Population Census, 1998. Islamabad, Pakistan: Ministry of Economic Affairs and Statistics, Government of Pakistan, 1998. http://www.statpak.gov.pk/depts/pco/statistics/statistics.html (accessed May 06, 08).

163. Ibid., ref. no. 132.

164. State Bank of Pakistan. Annual report of the State Bank of Pakistan, 2007. Islamabad, Pakistan: Government of Pakistan, 2008. http://www.sbp.org.pk/reports/annual/arfy07/index.htm (accessed Jan. 02, 09).

165. *Punjab, North West Frontier Province (NWFP), Sindh, Balochistan.*

166. *Federally Administered Tribal Areas (FATA); Federally Administered Northern Areas (FANA), Azad Jammu and Kashmir (AJK); and Islamabad Capital Territory (ICT).*

167. Ordinance Number VI of 2001: Government of Pakistan. Local Government Ordinance, 2001. http://www.nrb.gov.pk/publications/SBNP_Local_Govt_Ordinance_2001.pdf (accessed May 30, 08).

168. Fauji Foundation institutions, Pakistan. http://www.fauji.org.pk/Webforms/OurOrganization.aspx?Id=75 (accessed May 30, 08).

169. Federal Bureau of Statistics, Statistics Division. Pakistan Social and Living Standards Measurement Survey 2006-07. Islamabad, Pakistan: Government of Pakistan. http://www.statpak.gov.pk/depts/fbs/statistics/PSLSM2006_07/PSLSM2006_07.html (accessed April 30, 08).

170. Ibid., ref. no. 7.

171. Health Management and Information System; Ministry of Health, Government of Pakistan. http://www.pakistan.gov.pk/divisions/ContentInfo.jsp?DivID=25&cPath=254_260&ContentID=1635 (accessed May 08, 09).

172. Ministry of Population Welfare, Government of Pakistan. http://www.mopw.gov.pk/ (accessed Sep. 10, 08).

173. Ministry of Health, Government of Pakistan. http://www.health.gov.pk/ (accessed Sep 10. 08).

174. List of Hospitals in Pakistan. http://en.wikipedia.org/wiki/List_of_hospitals_in_Pakistan (accessed April 03, 09).

175. Gater R, de Almeida e Sousa B, Barrientos G, Caraveo J, Chandra Shekar CR, Dhadphale M, et al. The pathways to psychiatric care: a cross-cultural study. *Psychol Med* 1991;21(3):761-74.

176. Edhi Foundation. http://www.edhifoundation.com/ (accessed May 05, 09).

177. Rahnuma, Family Planning Association of Pakistan. http://www.fpapak.org/ (accessed Jan. 02, 09).

178. LUMS-McGill Social Enterprise Development Centre. Lahore, Pakistan: Lahore University of Management Sciences, 2005.

179. Ibid., ref. no. 7.

180. Ibid., ref. no. 34.

181. Ibid., ref. no. 143.

182. Ibid., ref. no. 144.

183. Mahbub-ul-Haq Human Development Centre. Human Development in South Asia 2007. Islamabad, Pakistan. Oxford University Press, 2008.

184. Nishtar S. Pakistan, politics and polio. *Bull World Health Organ* 2009 (Forthcoming).

185. Personal Communication. Executive Director, Pakistan Medical Research Council; April 07, 09. Unpublished results of the recently concluded National Survey for Hepatitis Prevalence, 2008. Pakistan Medical Research Council, Ministry of Health; Islamabad, Pakistan.

186. National AIDS Control Programme. National Study of Reproductive Tract Infections—Survey of High Risk Groups in Lahore and Karachi. Islamabad, Pakistan: Ministry of Health, Government of Pakistan, 2004.

187. National AIDS Control Programme. Pilot study under the HIV/AIDS Surveillance Project. Islamabad, Pakistan: Ministry of Health, Government of Pakistan, 2005.

188. Ibid., ref. no. 62.

189. Ministry of Finance. Poverty Reduction Strategy Paper 11. Islamabad, Pakistan: Ministry of Finance, Government of Pakistan, 2009. http://www.finance.gov.pk/admin/images/poverty/PRSP-II.pdf (accessed March 11, 09).

190. Planning Commission and UNICEF. National Nutritional Survey of West Pakistan, 2001-02. Islamabad, Pakistan: Government of Pakistan, 2002.

191. World Food Programme. WFP's Operational Requirements, Shortfalls and Priorities for 2008. http://www.documents.wfp.org/stellent/groups/public/documents/op_reports/wfp110572.pdf (accessed May 08, 08).

192. Vian T. Review of corruption in the health sector: theory, methods and interventions. *Health Policy Plan* 2008;23:83-94.

193. Transparency International. Global Corruption Report 2007. Transparency International, 2007. http://www.transparency.org/publications/gcr (accessed July 11, 08).

194. Gupta S, Davoodi H, Tiongron E. Corruption and the provision of healthcare and education services: Working Paper 00/116. Washington DC: International Monetary Fund, 2000. http://www.imf.org/external/pubs/ft/wp/2000/wp00116.pdf (accessed April 07, 09).

195. Azfar O. Corruption and the delivery of health and education services. Chapter 12 In: Spector BI, editor. Fighting Corruption in Developing Countries. Bloomfield, CT: Kumarian Press; 2005.

196. The World Bank. Country Policy and Institutional Assessment Measure. Washington DC, USA: The World Bank, 2006.

197. Ibid., ref. no. 193.

198. Gallup Pakistan. A survey on corruption in Pakistan. http://www.gallup.com.pk/pollsshow.php?id=2007-07-20 (accessed July 11, 08).

199. Pakistan Institute for Developmental Economics. Working paper 4 of 2006. Perception survey of the performance of civil servants in Pakistan. Islamabad, Pakistan: PIDE; 2006.

200. Transparency International. Corruption in South Asia—Insights and Benchmarks from Citizen Feedback Surveys in Five Countries. 2006.

201. Transparency International. Corruption in public services; informal payments among users of health services. Berlin, Germany: Transparency International; 2002.

202. Ibid., ref. no. 78.

203. Ibid., ref. no. 143.

204. Pakistan Council of Water Resources. Ministry of Science and Technology Government of Pakistan Islamabad. http://www.pcrwr.gov.pk/wq_phase2_report/wq_phase2_introduction.htm (accessed Dec. 05, 07).

205. Pakistan Medical Research Council and Statistics Division. National Health Survey of Pakistan 1992. Islamabad, Pakistan: Ministry of Health and Federal Bureau of Statistics, Government of Pakistan, 1992.

206. Anonymous. A country on the brink. *The Economist* 2008; 5-11:21-3.

207. Ibid., ref. no. 184.

208. Fikree F, Karim MS, Midhet F, Brendes HW. Causes of reproductive age mortality in low socioeconomic settlements in Karachi. *J Pak Med Assoc* 1993;43(10):208-12.

209. Midhet F, Becker S, Brendes HW. Contextual determinants of maternal mortality in rural Pakistan. *Soc Sci Med* 1998;46(12):1587-98.

210. Ibid., ref. no. 4.

211. Public Sector Group, Poverty Reduction and Economic Management Network. Reforming public institutions and strengthening governance: A World Bank strategy. Washington, D.C: The World Bank; 2000. http://www1.worldbank.org/publicsector/Reforming.pdf (accessed July 17, 08).

212. Kaufmann D, Kraay A, Lobaton PZ. Governance matters: Working Paper No. 2196. World Bank Policy Research Department. Washington DC, USA: The World Bank; 1999.

213. Travis P, Egger D, Davies P, Mechbal A. Towards better stewardship: concepts and critical issues. Geneva, Switzerland: World Health Organization, 2002. http://ww.who.int/whosis/discussion_papers/pdf/paper48.pdf (accessed July 17, 08).

214. Brinkerhoff DW, Bossert TJ. Health governance: concepts, experience and programming options for health systems 2020. Washington, DC: United States Agency for International Development, 2008.

215. Development Programme. Governance for Sustainable Human Development: a UNDP Policy Document. New York, UNDP, 1997. http://www.pogar.org/publications/other/undp/governance/undppolicydoc97-e.pdf (accessed April 07, 09).

216. Ibid., ref. no. 72.

217. Ibid., ref. no. 73.

218. Siddiqui S, Masud TI, Nishtar S, Peters DH, Sabri B, Bile KM, Jama MA. Framework for assessing governance of the health system in developing countries: Gateway to good governance. *Health Policy* 2008. [Epub ahead of print]

219. Ibid., ref. no. 214.

220. World Health Organization. Stewardship. http://www.who.int/healthsystems/stewardship/en/index.html (accessed May 26, 09).

221. Rowbottom R, Billis D. Organizational design: the work-levels approach. Aldershot: Gower; 1987.

222. Government of Pakistan. National Reconstruction Bureau. http://www.nrb.gov.pk/local_government/default.asp (accessed July 28, 08).

223. Ibid., ref. no. 167.

224. Pakistan Electronic Media Regulatory Authority. http://www.pemra.gov.pk/ (accessed April 07, 09).

225. *Population estimates based on the 1998 Population Census projections.*

226. Amin RA, Hay R. Health service costs and financing options for North West Frontier Province. Oxford, UK: Oxford Policy Management, 2002.

227. Ministry of Health and Population, Malawi. The Malawi Essential Health Package. http://www.sdnp.org.mw/~caphill/health/health1.htm (accessed Feb. 26, 08).

228. Tangcharoensathien V, Palu T. Primary health care: past achievements and future challenges, five country case studies. In: Three decades of primary health care: reviewing the past and defining the future; Bangkok, Thailand: Proceedings of the Prince Mahidol Award Conference, Jan 31-Feb 01; 2008.

229. Commission on Macroeconomics and Health. Investing in Health for Economic Development. Geneva, Switzerland: World Health Organization, 2001.

230. Fiscal Responsibility and Debt Limitation Act of Pakistan, 2005; (Act VI of 2005). http://www.finance.gov.pk/frdlo.pdf (accessed May 30, 08).

231. Debt Policy Coordination Office (DPCO), Ministry of Finance. Fiscal policy statement, 2008-09. Islamabad, Pakistan: Government of Pakistan, 2009. http://www.finance.gov.pk/admin/images/publications/Fiscal_Policy_Statement.pdf (accessed May 22, 09).

232. Finance Division, Government of Pakistan. Federal budget 2009-2010. Islamabad: Government of Pakistan; 2009.

233. Ibid., ref. no. 82.

234. McCoy D. The High Level Taskforce on Innovative International Financing for Health Systems. *Health Policy Plan* 2009;24: 321-3.

235. The Global Fund to Fight AIDS TB and Malaria. Innovative Financing. www.theglobalfund.org/en/funds_raised/innovative_financing/ (accessed Oct. 21, 08).

236. Ibid., ref. no. 143.

237. Federal Bureau of Statistics, Statistics Division. Respective Demographic Surveys for the years 1992-2003. Islamabad, Pakistan:. Government of Pakistan. http://www.statpak.gov.pk/depts/fbs/statistics/pds2001/pds2001.html. (accessed July 18, 08)

238. The World Bank. Pakistan Towards a Health Sector Strategy. Washington, USA: Health Population and Nutrition Unit, South Asia Region, World Bank, 1998.

239. Federal Bureau of Statistics. National health Accounts 2005-06. http://www.statpak.gov.pk/depts/fbs/publications/national_health_account2005_06/National_Health_Accounts.pdf (accessed May 20, 09).

240. Development Assistance Database, Pakistan. http://www.dadpak.org/dad/ (accessed April 07, 09).

241. FoDP form multi-donor trust fund. Daily Times 2009, Sep. 25. http://www.dailytimes.com.pk/default.asp?page=2009%5C09%5C25%5Cstory_25-9-2009_pg1_1 (accessed Sep. 25, 09).

242. Kerry-Lugar bill passed by US Senate. Daily Times 2009, Sep. 25. http://www.dailytimes.com.pk/default.asp?page=2009%5C09%5C25%5Cstory_25-9-2009_pg1_2 (accessed Sep. 25, 09).

243. Organization for Economic Cooperation and Development. Better Aid: 2008 Survey on Monitoring the Paris Declaration—Making Aid More Effective by 2010. ISBN 978-9264-05082-2. http://www.oecd.org/site/0,3407,en_21571361_39494699_1_1_1_1_1,00.html (accessed April 07, 09).

244. Ibid., ref. no. 239.

245. Nishtar S, Bile KM, Ahmed A, Amjad S, Iqbal A. Integrated population-based surveillance of non-communicable diseases the Pakistan model. *Am J Prev Med* 2005;29(5 Suppl 1):102-6.

246. Siddiqa A. Military Inc.: Inside Pakistan's Military Economy. Karachi, Pakistan: Oxford University Press; 2007.

247. Pakistan Centre for Philanthropy. Bridging the Gap for Social Development. http://www.pcp.org.pl/fact_sheet.html (accessed Sep. 25, 09).

248. CGI Member Commitments. Heartfile: Using technology to promote equity in health financing, 2008. www.clintonglobalinitiative.org/NETCOMMUNITY/Page.aspx?pid=2612&srcid=2605 (accessed Feb. 09).

249. *Computation of pooling takes into account contributions of Fauji Foundation, the Employees Social Security Institute, Autonomous Agencies, as well as the corporate sector and philanthropy.*

250. Ibid., ref. no. 142.

251. Takaful Pakistan Limited. http://www.takaful.com.pk/HealthPolicy.html (accessed Sep. 1, 09).

252. Ministry of Religious Affairs. Concept of Zakat. Government of Pakistan. http://www.pakistan.gov.pk/ministries/religious-affairs-ministry/media/ZakatCollectionandDistributionSystem.doc (accessed June 11, 08).

253. Ministry of Labour, Manpower and Overseas Pakistanis. Informal Sector-Zakat. In: Social Protection Strategy Development Study, Final Report Vol. I: Social Protection. Asian Development Bank, 2008. http://www.adb.org/Documents/Reports/Consultant/37008-PAK/vol1/chap4.pdf (accessed June 11, 08).

254. Ibid., ref. no. 138.

255. Benazir Income Support Programme. http://www.bisp.gov.pk/benazir/ (accessed May 06, 09).

256. Lagomarsino G, Kundra SS. Risk Pooling: Challenges and Opportunities. Washington, USA: Results for Development; 2008.

257. Ibid.

258. Ibid., ref. no. 138.

259. Ibid.

260. Ibid., ref. no. 140.

261. Ibid., ref. no. 139.

262. Ibid., ref. no. 248.

263. Ibid. ref. no. 104.

264. England R. Provider purchasing and contracting mechanisms: better understanding the role of the private sector in health systems: challenges and opportunities. Rockefeller Foundation and HLSP institute. London: 2008.

265. Rwanda. Performance-based financing in health. Third International Roundtable Source Book. http://www.managingfordevelopmentresults.org/Sourcebook/pdf/3cRwanda.pdf (accessed April 21, 08).

266. Eichler R, Auxila P, Pollock J. Output based health care: paying for performance in Haiti. The World Bank Group; Private Sector and Infrastructure Network. Viewpoint no 236, Aug 2001. http://www-wds.worldbank.org/ (accessed March 20, 08).

267. Ibid., ref. no. 143.

268. Lewis M. Informal Health Payments in Central and Eastern Europe and the Former Soviet Union: Issues, Trends and Policy Implications. In: Funding Health Care: Option for Europe. Figuers and Moussiales, editors. Buckingham, UK: Open University Press, 2002.

269. Ministry of Health. Health legislation on the Anvil. Islamabad, Pakistan: Government of Pakistan, 2000.

270. United States Agency for International Aid and Pakistan Initiative for Mothers and Newborns. Functional Integration of Services, Rawalpindi District Pilot Study. Islamabad, Pakistan: JSI-PAIMAN, 2007.

271. Ibid., ref. no. 15.

272. Ibid., ref. no. 61.

273. Ibid., ref. no. 169.

274. Ibid., ref. no. 149.

275. Canadian International Development Agency. Community Information and Epidemiological Technology. http://www.ciet.org/en/aboutciet/ (accessed Aug. 06, 08).

276. Federal Bureau of Statistics, Statistics Division. Pakistan Integrated Household Survey 2001-02. Islamabad, Pakistan: Government of Pakistan, 2001.

277. Punjab Rural Support Programme. Government of Punjab, Pakistan. http://www.prsp.org.pk/ (accessed July 11, 08).

278. Ibid., ref. no. 25.

279. Ibid., ref. no. 106.

280. Amjad S. Review and assessment of Primary Health Care models in Pakistan. Study Commissioned by USAID: in press, 2009.

281. Ibid.

282. Toll K, Agha S. Country Watch: Pakistan. *Sex Health Exch* 1999;1:7-8.

283. Oxford Policy Management. Lady Health Worker Programme's external evaluation of the National Programme for Family Planning and Primary Health Care: NWFP and FATA survey report. London, UK: Oxford Policy Management; 2002.

284. Federal Bureau of Statistics, Statistics Division Pakistan Integrated Household Survey. Islamabad, Pakistan: Government of Pakistan, 2002.

285. Ibid., ref. no. 144.

286. Federal Programme Implementation Unit. Field program officers' survey 2007: Internal assessment of Lady Health Worker Programme. Islamabad, Pakistan: Ministry of Health, Government of Pakistan, 2007.

287. Nishtar S. The Gateway Paper—preventive and promotive programs in Pakistan and health reforms in Pakistan. *J Pak Med Assoc* 2006 Dec;56(12 Suppl. 4):S51-65.

288. Afsar HA, Yunus M. Recommendations to strengthen the role of LHWs in the National Programme for Family Planning and Primary Health Care in Pakistan: the health workers perspective. *J Ayub Med Coll Abbottabad* 2005;17(1):48-53.

289. Afsar HA, Qureshi AF, Younis M, Gulb A, Mahmood A. Factors affecting unsuccessful referral by the lady health workers in Karachi, Pakistan. *J Pak Med Assoc* 2003;53:521.

290. Ibid., ref. no. 107.

291. Ibid., ref. no. 53.

292. Nishtar S, Amjad S, Sheikh S, Ahmed M. Synergizing health and population in Pakistan. *J Pak Med Assoc* 2009;59 (9 suppl.3).

293. Liu X, Hotchkiss DR, Bose S, Bitran R, Giedon U. Contracting for primary health services: evidence on its effects and a framework for evaluation. Bethesda (MD): Partnerships for Health Reform Project, Abt Associates Inc; 2004.

294. Ibid., ref. no. 125.

295. Ibid., ref. no. 126.

296. David MC, Zeckhauser RJ. The Anatomy of Health Insurance. In: Culyer AJ and Newhouse JP, editors. Handbook of health economics, Volume I. Amsterdam: Elsevier; 563-643.

297. Prahalad CK. The fortune at the bottom of the pyramid. Eradicating poverty through profits. New Jersey, USA: Wharton school publishing; 2004.

298. Shah J, Murty LS. Compassionate, High Quality Care at Low Cost: The Aravind Model. IIMB *Management Review* 2004;16(3).

299. Mackie S, Misra R, Sharma A, Prahalad CK. Jaipur Foot: Challenging Convention. University of Michigan Business School; 2003.

300. Khanna T, Rangan KV, Manocaran M. Narayan Hrudayalaya Heart Hospital: Cardiac Care for the Poor. Boston: Harvard Business Publishing; 2006. Report No: 9-505-078.

301. Gwatkin DR. Reducing health Inequalities in developing countries. In: Detels R, McEven J, Beaglehole R, Tanaka H, editors. Oxford Textbook of Public Health.4th ed. Oxford: Oxford University Press; 2002.

302. International trade, trade agreements, and health: implications on Primary Health Care. In: Three Decades of Primary Health Care: Reviewing the past and defining the future. Prince Mahidol Award Conference 2008. http://www.pmaconference.org/index.php?option=com_content&task=view&id=49&Itemid=74 (accessed June 17, 08).

303. Rizvi SA, Naqvi SA, Zafar MN, Mazhar F, Muzaffar R, Naqvi R, Akhtar F, Ahmed E. Commercial transplants in local Pakistanis from vended kidneys: a socio-economic and outcome study. *Transpl Int* 2009;22(6):615-21.(7)2009 Jan 31. [Epub ahead of print].

304. Nishtar S. Legislative Brief: Transplantation of Human Organs and Tissues Bill. Islamabad, Pakistan: Pakistan Institute of Legislative Development and Transparency, 2007. http://www.pildat.org/search.asp?q=Nishtar+S&B1=+&sitesearch=http%3A%2F%2Fwww.pildat.org&domains=http%3A%2F%2Fwww.pildat.org&ie=UTF-8&oe=UTF-8 (accessed June 17, 08).

305. Personal Communication. Pakistan Nursing Council; January 2008.

306. Bossert T. Decentralization of health systems: decision space, innovation, and performance. Holyoke, Cambridge MA: Harvard School of Public Health; 1998. http://www.hsph.harvard.edu/ihsg/publications/pdf/No-54.PD (accessed July 24, 08).

307. Ibid., ref. no. 129

308. World Health Organization. The World Health Report 2006: Working Together For Health. Geneva, Switzerland: WHO, 2006. http://www.who.int/whr/2006/06_overview_en.pdf (accessed July 01, 08).

309. Ibid., ref. no. 78.

310. Ibid., ref. no. 149.

311. Higher Education Commission, Government of Pakistan. Model track process statutes, 2008. http://www.hec.gov.pk/QualityAssurance/QA_Agency/Tenure_Track.htm (accessed July 24, 08).

312. Ibid., ref. no. 155.

313. National Commission for Government reforms. National training strategy for civil services: working paper for the 2nd meeting of the Steering Committee. Islamabad, Pakistan: Establishment Division, Government of Pakistan, 2007. http://www.ncgr.gov.pk/All_Reforms_Papers.html (accessed March 14, 08).

314. Ibid., ref. no. 8.

315. Cockburn R, Newton PN, Agyarko K, Akunyili D, White NJ. The global threat of counterfeit drugs: Why industry and governments must communicate the dangers. http://www.plosmedicine.org/article/info:doi/10.1371/journal.pmed.0020100 (accessed May 07, 09).

316. Ibid., ref. no. 146.

317. Personal communication. Drug Controller; Ministry of Health, Pakistan. January 2009: unpublished data.

318. Ibid.

319. World Health Organization. Resolution # WHA 56.27 dated May 28, 2003. Intellectual Property Rights, Innovation and Public Health. http://www.who.int/gb/ebwha/pdf_files/WHA56/ea56r27.pdf (accessed July 31, 08).

320. Doha Declaration on the TRIPS Agreement and Public Health http://www.wto.org/english/theWTO_e/minist_e/min01_e/mindecl_trips_e.htm (accessed July 31, 08).

321. Tantivess S, Terrawattanon S, Mohara A. Assessing the implications of Thailand's government use licenses, issued in 2006-08. Nonthaburi: Thailand, Health Intervention Technology Assessment Program, 2009. http://hitap.net/backoffice/news/news_display2_en.php/=3750 (accessed Sep. 26, 09).

322. Agreement on Trade related Aspects of Intellectual Property Rights Annex 1C, Art 28 (entered into force 1994) http://www.wtc.org/english/tratop_e/trips_e/t_agm2_e.htm (accessed July 31, 08).

323. Pakistan Telecommunication Authority. http://www.pta.gov.pk (accessed May 20, 09).

324. Personal Communication. M. Tariq Badsha; Technology Consultant to Heartfile. May 10, 2009.

325. Planning Commission, Government of Pakistan. Social Development: Information technology & telecommunications division; Public Sector Development Programmes, 2009-10. http://115.186.133.3/pcportal/psdp/PSDP%202009-10/IT%20and%20Telecom.pdf (accessed Sep. 26, 09).

326. Rashid E, Ishtiaq O, Gilani S, Zafar A. Comparison of store and forward method of teledermatology with face-to-face consultation. *J Ayub Med Coll Abbottabad*. 2003 Apr-Jun;15(2):34-6.

327. Zafar A, Belard JL, Gilani S, Murad F, Khan M, Merrell RC. The impact of curriculum on a national telehealth program. *Telemed J E Health.* 2008 Mar;14(2):195-8.

328. Meade K, Lam DM. A deployable telemedicine capability in support of humanitarian operations. *Telemed J E Health* 2007;13(3):331-40.

329. Gul S, Ghaffar H, Mirza S, Fizza Tauqir S, Murad F, Ali Q, Zafar Malik A, Merrell RC. Multitasking a telemedicine training unit in earthquake disaster response: paraplegic rehabilitation assessment. *Telemed J E Health* 2008;14(3):280-3.

330. Telehealth project in Northern Pakistan. http://technhealth.blogspot.com/2007/04/telehealth-project-in-northern-pakistan.html (accessed Feb. 12, 09).

331. Ibid., ref. no. 248.

332. Khoja S, Scott R, Gilani S. E-health readiness assessment: promoting "hope" in the health-care institutions of Pakistan. *World Hosp Health Serv* 2008;44(1):36-8.

333. Ibid., ref. no. 143.

334. Ibid.

335. The World Bank. Public health surveillance system: a call for action. Islamabad, Pakistan: Ministry of Health, World Bank, Centres for Disease Control, World Health Organization; 2005.

336. Ministry of Health. Infectious disease surveillance plan. Islamabad, Pakistan: National Institute of Health; 2005.

337. Center for Disease Control and Prevention. Field Epidemiology and Laboratory Training Programme. http://islamabad.usembassy.gov/pakistan/h06091601.html (accessed July 01, 08).

338. Ibid., ref. no. 245.

339. Heartfile. Surveillance: National Action Plan for Prevention and Control of Non-Communicable Diseases and Health Promotion in Pakistan; Heartfile. http://heartfile.org/napsurv.htm (accessed Dec. 11, 08).

340. Japan International Cooperation Agency HMIS Study Team. National Action Plan. In: The study of improvement of management information systems in the health sector in Pakistan. Pakistan: Scientific System Consultants (Japan), Pakistan Ministry of Health, JICA; 2006

341. Ibid., ref. no. 144.

342. World Health Organization. Pakistan Global Youth Tobacco Survey (GYTS) 2003. http://apps.who.int/infobase/reportviewer.aspx?rptcode=ALL&uncode=586&dm=8&surveycode=102547b1 (accessed May 20, 09).

343. Commission on Human Security. Human Security Now. New York, USA; United Nations, 2003. http://www.humansecurity-chs.org/finalreport/English/FinalReport.pdf (accessed April 07, 09).

344. Nishtar S. Nuancing national security. The News International 2009 August 22; sect. comment:6. http://www.thenews.com.pk/print1.asp?id=194209(accessed Sep. 26, 09).

345. Frenk J. Health Security for All: A Comprehensive Focus for Health System Strengthening. International Conference on Global Action for Health System Strengthening. Tokyo, Japan. November 3-4, 2008.

346. Weekly Epidemiological Records, October 3, 2008, World Health Organization. Human cases of Avian influenza-A (H5N1) in NWFP, Pakistan during the period October-November 2007. http://www.who.int/wer/2008/wer8340.pdf (accessed April 07, 09).

347. The United Nations Convention against Corruption United Nations General Assembly (Resolution 58/4). 2003. http://www.en.wikipedia.org/wiki/United_Nations_Convention_against_Corruption (accessed July18, 08).

348. Nishtar S. Institutionalizing accountability. The NEWS International 2009, May 25; sect. comment:6. http://www.thenews.com.pk/arc_news.asp?id=9(accessed Sep. 26, 09).

349. Ibid., ref. no. 188.

350. Commission on the Social Determinants of Health (CSDH). Achieving Health Equity: from root causes to fair outcomes—interim Statement. Geneva, Switzerland: World Health Organization, 2007. http://whqlibdoc.who.int/publications/2007/interim_statement_eng.pdf (accessed June 23, 08).

351. Kaber N. Gender Equality and Human Development: The Instrumental rationale. Brighton, UK: United Nation Development Programme, 2005. http://www.hdr.undp.org/en/reports/global/hdr2005/papers/hdr2005_kabeer_naila_31.pdf (accessed June 25, 08).

352. Pakistan Council of Research in Water Resources. Ministry of Science and Technology. Government of Pakistan Islamabad. http://www.pcrwr.gov.pk/wq_phase2_report/wq_phase2_introduction.htm (accessed June 23, 08).

353. Ibid., ref. no. 205.

354. Xu K, Evans DB, Kawabata K, Zeramdini R, Klavus J, Murray C. Household catastrophic health expenditure: a multi-country Analysis. *Lancet* 2003, 362, 111-7.

355. Ibid., ref. no. 138.

356. Gish O. Brain Drain. The Nation, Lahore 1997, Nov 13. http://meltingpot.fortunecity.com/botswana/616/oscar.html (accessed June 25, 08).

357. Syed R. Pharma exports to touch $600m by 2010. Daily Times 2007, June 30. http://www.dailytimes.com.pk/default.asp?page=2007\06\30\story_30-6-2007_pg5_2 (accessed June 23, 08).

358. Nishtar S. What is the role of the state in health? The NEWS International 2007, Feb 25; sect. comment:6. http://heartfile.org/pdf/19_M-Tower.pdf (accessed June 23, 08).

359. Ibid., ref. no. 138.

360. Ibid., ref. no. 255.

361. Issues and Policies Consultants. Pakistan: Review of selected social safety net programs. Issues and Policies Consultants; Lahore, Pakistan, 2004.

362. The World Bank. South Asia: Data Projects and Research, 2008. http://web.worldbank.org/WBSITE/EXTERNAL/COUNTRIES/SOUTHASIAEXT/0,pagePK:158889~piPK:146815~theSitePK:223547,00.html (accessed June 23, 08).

363. Nishtar S. Pakistan's covert cartels. The NEWS International 2008, May 22; sect.comment:6. http://heartfile.org/pdf/29_CovertCartels.pdf (accessed June 10, 08).

364. Nishtar S. Social Policy Reform—raison d' etre. Blue Chip: January, 2007. http://heartfile.org/pdf/18_datre.pdf (accessed June 02, 08).

365. Ministry of Health, Government of Pakistan. National Health Policy 2001: The Way Forward. Agenda for Health Sector Reform http://siteresources.worldbank.org/PAKISTANEXTN/Resources/Pakistan-Development-Forum/NationalHealthPolicy.pdf (accessed May 07, 09).

366. Ibid., ref. no. 78.

367. Ibid., ref. no. 9.

368. Heartfile. Post-Gateway Policy Roundtables. http://heartfile.org/pgpr.htm (accessed April 08, 08).

369. Ibid., ref. no. 80.

370. Ibid., ref. no. 84.

371. Buse K, Mays N, Walt G. Making Health Policy. Milton Keynes, UK: Open University Press. 2005.

372. Ibid., ref. no. 143.

373. Nishtar S. Honing the 100-day agenda. The NEWS International 2008, April 06; sect. comment:6. http://heartfile.org/pdf/28_100-day_agenda.pdf (accessed June10, 08).

374. Ibid., ref. no. 85.

375. Ibid., ref. no. 167.

376. Ibid., ref. no. 144.

377. Ibid., ref. no. 292.

378. World Health Organization. Ottawa Charter for Health Promotion. Ottawa, Canada: World Health Organization, 1986. http://en.wikipedia.org/wiki/Ottawa_Charter_for_Health_Promotion (accessed Aug. 04, 08).

379. Department of legal and legislative affairs, Punjab. The Punjab infrastructure (development and regulation) Amendment act (Punjab Act No. 22 of 2003) Punjab Govt. gaz. (extra), (kRTK12, 1925 SAKA) Islamabad, Pakistan; 2003. prbdb.gov.in/files/Acts/PIDB%20Amendment%20Ac (accessed July 04, 08).

380. Halsbury's Laws of India, Volume 29(1), Butterworths India 2001 at 285.001

381. Donoghue v. Stevenson [1932] AC 562 (House of Lords).

382. Punjab Road Transport Corporation v. Zahida Afzal and Others [2006 SCMR 207], per Tassaduq Hussain Jillani, J. p. 215.

383. Alia Tareen v. Amanullah Khan, Advocate [PLD 2005 Supreme Court 99].

384. Ibid., ref. no. 381.

385. International Monetary Fund. IMF Executive Board Concludes 2009 Article IV Consultation with Pakistan; Public Information Notice (PIN) No. 09/43

April 3, 2009. http://www.imf.org/external/np/sec/pn/2009/pn0943.htm (accessed May 20, 09).

386. APC endorsed Swat offensive The NEWS International 2009, May 18. http://www.thenews.com.pk/updates.asp?id=78037 (accessed May 20, 09).

387. Ibid., ref. no. 62.

Acknowledgements

The background research for this publication was carried out at Heartfile—the NGO think tank that I founded in 1999. As such, therefore, I am indebted to several members of my team for their help with retrieving documents and information and helping with computations.

I am thankful to Yasir Abbas Mirza and Faraz Khalid for their help with following up requests for information from various sources and helping with managing excel sheets and carrying out the computations. I am thankful to Saba Amjad for formatting and archiving references and to Amina Katrina Ronis and Sohail Amjad for their comments on various sections. I am also thankful to Azhar Iqbal, Amjad Javed and Aamra Qayyum for lending administrative support within the organization.

A number of colleagues outside of the organization provided comments on various sections. In this regard, I am thankful to Hans V. Hogerzeil, Farid Khan and Ghalib Nishtar for their comments on the Chapter on *Medicines and Related Products*; Tariq Badsha for his comments on the Chapter on *Technology in Health Systems*; Bernt Struck for his comments on the Chapter on *Health Financing*; Sikandar Bashir Mohmand for his review of the section on *Personal and product liability litigation and legislation* and Ties Boerma for his comments on the Chapter on *Health Information Systems.*

I am thankful to Shahina Maqbool for her help with conforming the manuscript with the style sheet of the publisher and for proof reading the manuscript in the end and Zulfiqar Ali for layout designing of the manuscript.

I am also very grateful to Ghousia Ali, Managing Editor, Oxford University Press for her help with the process that led to the publication of the manuscript and Professor Julio Frenk for agreeing to write the foreword of the book.

My family deserves my gratitude for the support that enables me to fulfill my pursuits. My mother Tahira Hamid's blessings; my mother-in-law Riffat Nishtar's support; my husband Ghalib Nishtar's encouragement and my children Kassim and Leena's affection has been a source of great support for me. The memory of my late father's values continues to be a source of inspiration, for which I am eternally grateful.

Finally, I am thankful to all those colleagues and friends around the world, discussions with whom have helped me hone my understanding about the complexity of health systems.

Sania Nishtar

Appendix

The Gateway Health Policy Scaffold

The Vision

A new vision for the health sector involves organizing the future health system to deliver on the Health for All premise in line with contemporary realities—a strong and resilient health system that:

- Addresses social inequities and inequities in health and is fair, responsive, and pro-poor;
- Supports people and communities to attain the highest possible level of health and well-being;
- Reduces excess mortality, morbidity, and disability and caregivers burden—especially in poor and marginalized populations;
- Mitigates risks to health that arise from environmental, economic, social, and behavioural causes;
- Meets the specific needs of health promotion as well as treatment, prevention, and control of diseases; and
- Is there when you need it—a health system that encourages you to have your say and ensures that your views are taken into account.

The principles that support this vision state:

that all men and women should have EQUITABLE opportunities to improve and maintain their well-being;

that mitigating social inequities and achieving SOCIAL JUSTICE is fundamental to improving health outcomes, given the strong correlation between social inequities and health inequalities;

that priorities for the use of public funds and the criteria for setting those PRIORITIES should be PEOPLE-CENTRED;

that an INTER-SECTORAL APPROACH to health, which seeks to coordinate and streamline policies and actions within the health sector with other sectors, integrating relevant economic, developmental, political, socio-cultural, trade, environmental, and national security related concerns into health systems planning is critical to improving health outcomes;

that GENDER MAINSTREAMING and COMMUNITY EMPOWERMENT in planning and implementation of all health programmes will reduce gender disparities and increase acceptance;

that UNIVERSAL COVERAGE for a basic set of health interventions is a fundamental responsibility of the state and should be provided for all without economic, geographical, social, or cultural barriers;

that EVIDENCE-BASED DECISION-MAKING must prevail at every level of the health system so that policy development and actions deriving from policies are relevant, sustainable, feasible, resource appropriate, and culturally and socially acceptable;

that a paradigm shift from a planning environment concentrated on the reporting of processes and outputs to OUTCOME ORIENTATION will improve health outcomes;

that FAIR FINANCING can make the delivery of services more equitable and outcome oriented;

that a focus on QUALITY MANAGEMENT by the government will ensure safe and patient-centred delivery of high quality healthcare;

that various levels of the health system in the private and public sectors need to be strengthened and linked in order to be able to deliver the most appropriate level of care, and that health system investments need to follow the principle of SUBSIDIARITY in order to make them more efficient, responsive, and sustainable and that the hallmarks of this approach include devolution, impact orientation, and transparency in governance;

that TECHNICAL EFFICIENCY, which is concerned with the production of services at minimum cost; and ALLOCATIVE EFFICIENCY, which is concerned with producing the right collection of outputs is important for achieving health systems objectives.

The broad goals of the new vision and the envisaged agenda for policy reform and their respective strategies fall within the following eight domains:

- Evidence and information
- Health in all policies
- Health promotion
- Leadership and governance
- Health financing
- Service delivery
- Health workforce
- Medicines, products, and technologies

1. Evidence and information

Evidence must form the basis of decision-making relevant to any area in the health sector—promotive, preventive, therapeutic, rehabilitative, or management related.

Goal: to garner an unyielding political and institutional commitment to base decisions on evidence and institutionalize rational accountability of the decision-making process; and to develop a sustainable health information infrastructure and capacity within the health system to systematically collect, consolidate, analyze, and interpret health data and information, and relay it in a timely manner for actions at appropriate levels.

Strategies:

1. Strengthening the institutional pillars—a comprehensive *data and information policy*, ethical conduct in the data system, an *apex institutional arrangement* for the National Health Information System, a *mechanism to periodically report on health indicators and evidence*, and strategic investments in priority research areas from budgetary and extra-budgetary sources.

2. Strengthening the programme pillars—integration of piecemeal infectious disease surveillance activities into an integrated disease surveillance system; institutionalizing population-based surveillance of NCD risk factors; improving the cause of death system; bridging the weaknesses of the Health Management and Information System; developing methods, instruments, and measures for health systems, policy, and operational research; consolidating health and demographic survey capacity; establishing a national system for health surveys building on existing population-based instruments; and strengthening institutional mechanisms for research in academic and other relevant settings.

3. Building institutional capacity to comply with the stipulations of international health regulations and other globally binding arrangements.

4. Ensuring that data are disaggregated by income levels, districts, gender, and other socio-economic determinants in the data system in order to facilitate targeting of interventions to appropriate groups.

2. Health in all policies

Many factors influence and determine health at individual and population levels. The broader determinants of health can be socio-economic, environmental, and biological, or lifestyle related. Most, but not all of these, can be modified through action within or outside the health system—in case of the latter, within the broader inter-sectoral domain.

Goal: to regard health within an *inter-sectoral scope* in a broad national and international policy context; to ensure that people receive a clear benefit from the health system in terms of *health gains*, which are concerned with health status and *social gains, which are* concerned with broader aspects of quality of life; to support *vulnerable households* in managing hazards and risks and to build equity safeguards with respect to the emergence of health as a sector within the market economy.

Strategies

5. Pro-poor macroeconomic growth, which results in job creation and income supplementation of poor families.

6. Better macroeconomic management so that there is additional fiscal space to spend on health; financial sector reforms to expand the tax base; and legal and institutional measures for fiscal responsibility to limit debt, which constrains fiscal space, and fiscal transparency to minimize leakages from the system.

7. Formulating appropriate policies aimed at addressing *absolute deprivation* associated with low socio-economic status, *relative deprivation* or inequitable distribution of income, and *broader social inequalities* such as gender and geographic inequalities.

8. Broadening the base of social protection instruments—publicly funded safety nets, cash transfer schemes, and entitlements built into labour legislation—to protect the poor against health shocks.

9. Strengthening the government's redistributive role to build safeguards against the negative social impacts of policies in other sectors as the balance in the economy is pushed in the direction of public rather than private ownership.

10. Focusing on the scope of public health work conventionally placed outside of medical care service—provision of clean water and solid waste disposal.

11. Use of technology infrastructure and network connectivity for strengthening health information systems, disseminating information for behaviour change communication and capacity building, better targeting of programmes and subsidies, reducing costs and medical errors in health facilities, and promoting transparency within the health system.

12. Establishing linkages with ministries for action outside of the healthcare domain to improve health outcomes—*transport* (injury prevention); *agriculture* (food security, crop substitution, and agro-industrial diversification—the latter in the context of tobacco control); *Central Board of Revenue* (taxation and dependence on revenues generated from tobacco); *trade and commerce* (post-WTO concerns and counterfeiting of medicines); *Industries and Environment* (National Environmental Quality Standards); and *Narcotics Control Division* (substance abuse).

13. Collaboration with institutional arrangements for disaster management to ensure effective response in the case of conflicts, terrorism, global pandemics, natural disasters, humanitarian crises, and food insecurity.

3. Health promotion

Health promotion is a participatory empowering equity focused process—one that regards community participation as being essential to every stage of health promoting actions, as well as one that leverages community assets and knowledge to create the necessary conditions for health.

Goal: to enable people and communities to make appropriate use of health services and exercise control over their own health and well-being by ensuring their participation in decisions, which impact their quality of life.

Strategies:

14. Health promoting public policies, which create and promote supportive environments in schools, workplaces, health services, and the community in order to promote healthy behaviours.

15. Integration of environmental and occupational health within the ambit of public health with reference to the effects of urbanization, air, noise and chemical pollution, environmental degradation, and agricultural and industrial pollutants.

16. Focusing on lifestyle related preventable risks to health—promotion of physical activity, healthy eating, safe sexuality, cessation of tobacco use, curbing the use of illicit drugs, and promoting blood safety.

4. Leadership and governance

Issues of management and governance have been identified as one of the key impediments to leveraging the potential within Pakistan's extensive physical health infrastructure, and appear to be largely responsible for the poor health status of the country's population.

Goal: to enhance transparency, effectiveness, efficiency, and responsiveness in governance by improving accountability to the people, and to foster evidence-based decision-making as the norm.

Strategies:

17. Capacity building and reorientation of the role of the Ministry of Health to enable it to effectively perform its core normative

functions—information and evidence management, policy-making, developing a vision for reforming the sector, oversight, monitoring, assurance and regulation, economic coordination, ensuring compliance with international regulations, and providing overall leadership in the health sector in order to capitalize the strengths of all actors within the health system.

18. Capacity building and reorientation of the role of the departments of health to enable them to effectively oversee provision of and access to good quality healthcare for all, by the districts.

19. Enhancing leadership and management competencies of state functionaries through capacity building initiatives; and strengthening of the public management process through public sector and civil service reform for effective governance in the domains of implementation, oversight, and regulation.

20. Human resource policies on training, recruitment, retention, and deployment that incentivize and sustainably institutionalize individuals with competencies in health systems domains.

21. A result-based culture in governance, linking results to overall national goals and objectives and focusing on performance enhancement, both through the creation of an enabling milieu—market compatible incentives, building capacity and decentralizing decision-making and fiscal controls—as well as through the enhancement of accountability.

22. Effective devolution characterized by administrative and financial decentralization in line with the principles of subsidiarity, political and administrative ownership, clarity in roles, responsibilities, and prerogatives, grass roots empowerment, community oversight and strengthening of capacities for effective and equitable service delivery at the district level.

23. Structuring state and quasi-state organizational entities in a manner so that functions of policy-making, regulation, and implementation are clearly assigned to organizational entities. Granting administrative

and financial autonomy to organizational entities in line with the principles of subsidiarity.

24. Fostering greater inter-sectoral coordination at the federal, provincial, and district levels.

25. A policy shift in the health sector to additionally focus on population planning; functionally integrating the ministries of health and population and creating optimal synergies between the population and health programmes in order to address the high ratio of unmet need for family planning and improve reproductive health outcomes.

26. Support for broader transparency promoting *systemic technocratic and sectoral reform*—civil service reform, reform of public financial management, and procurement and audit systems. Advocacy for *overall structural changes within the state* so as to reform political institutions, strengthen systems of judicial redress and mechanisms of civil society oversight, ensure freedom of information and an open media, enable avenues for seeking redress, and promote economic reforms that weaken the concentration of organized economic vested interest.

27. Inculcating democratic behaviours at the individual and institutional levels in governance and institutionalizing democratic values of liberty, equality, freedom, and rights as an institutional norm.

5. Health financing

Health financing is the key tool in making the delivery of services more equitable and outcome-oriented.

Goal: to maximize public sources of health financing (revenues and social health insurance) over private sources (out-of-pocket payments and private insurance) and to enable universal coverage for a certain set of essential interventions through revenues and provide alternative means of health financing for achieving the equity objective.

Strategies

28. Enhancing government revenue expenditure on health to provide adequate financing for ensuring the delivery of essential services and promoting equitable allocation to ensure that a wider segment of the population benefits from higher public expenditures.

29. A focus on getting the best value for the government's investment in health by improving utilization of funds, addressing technical and allocative inefficiencies, rationalizing transaction costs, improving transparency in the management of resources, and ensuring better expenditure tracking.

30. Establishing an overarching mechanism to ensure that health allocations from the general revenue pool for the federal, provincial, and district levels are fully integrated and explicitly support a consistent and coherent set of nationally agreed objectives in line with stated priorities. Additionally, ensuring that there are mechanisms in place to evaluate the impact of given allocations on outcomes vis-à-vis the equity objective and the poverty reduction strategy focus.

31. Exerting influence on the districts to spend more and better on health to ensure the delivery of the essential health services package and using fiscal tools as incentives for this purpose.

32. Ensuring that development assistance is actually needed in the country; that it fulfils a strategic priority need; that it will predictably and reliably support country-led efforts and that it will have no explicit or implicit harmful effects in the county over the long term nor undermine the sustainability of programmes. Channelling development assistance to help strengthen systems with a view to ultimately transition away from such support; and promote debt forgiveness as a tool to free up resources for health and other social sectors.

33. Broadening the base of risk pooling for those in the formally employed sector through *insurance* and for those in the informally employed sector through *exemption* systems.

34. Incentivizing as well as making it binding for employers to subscribe to global employment practices and provide coverage to employees by pooling employers' as well as employees' contributions through payroll taxes, where feasible.

35. Broadening the base of pooling in existing social health insurance arrangements—vertically organized arrangements such as the Employees Social Security Institute and others—to cover a wider segment of low-income employees for health.

36. Incentivizing the current policy environment for private insurance companies and balancing financial incentives with appropriate safeguards and incentives for employers so as to encourage them to subscribe, whilst ensuring that measures help to decrease inequities.

37. Establishing health equity funds as part of social protection arrangements and using cash transfers through exemption systems as a targeting approach in order to protect the poor against catastrophic expenditure on health.

38. Collaborating with microfinance institutions to offset costs and risks involved in administering community health insurance schemes in far-flung areas by providing subsidies and underwriting costs.

39. Separation of the financing vis-à-vis service delivery roles of state agencies, where needed, on the premise that such separation can affect the performance of health facilities; institutionalizing purchasing of 'non-priority' high-cost curative services for disadvantaged groups to meet the equity objective.

40. Employing purchasing as a tool in public-private relationships and in government to public sector service delivery agency relationships to make service providers accountable for delivering specific and

measurable activities; utilizing performance based financing for improving service delivery outcomes.

6. Government services and facilities

The state has the mandate and responsibility to guide, oversee, and ensure the delivery of services to all its citizens on an equitable basis.

Goal: to ensure the delivery of quality essential services to all citizens leveraging the strength and outreach of *all* stakeholders in the health sector—both state as well as non-state.

Strategies:

41. Definition of essential services scoping beyond areas stipulated by the Millennium Development Goals, basing decisions on objective assessment of the burden of disease, and ensuring that neglected diseases and strategies are addressed.

42. Expanding the focus of Primary Health Care as a development concept and tool to encompass both the *set of activities and services to be delivered* as well as considerations relevant to *the first point of contact with individuals.* As a *set of services*, a locally developed MDG+ package needs to be used as a benchmark for publicly provided services and the basis of contractual relationships with non-state actors, when engaged to deliver services. As a *first point of contact,* a set of additional strategies should be employed to augment coverage of Primary Health Care by harnessing the potential of non-state actors to achieve universal coverage through publicly financed alternative delivery mechanisms. This can include contracting private providers in the short to medium term and training a cadre of family practitioners in the long term.

43. Integration of national public health programmes within the provincial-district accounting and accountability channels in order to address current issues created by multiple channels of accountability and management.

44. Restructuring management of public facilities while ensuring that the restructured system has checks and balances with designated roles for *management, quality assurance and evaluation,* and *community oversight;* that restructuring is need-based and strengthens decentralization and community oversight; and that the state does not divest from its core responsibilities in restructured management arrangements.

45. Enhancing capacities of, and empowering local governments to deploy locally-suited options for facility restructuring, albeit with appropriate safeguards; assisting with and enabling them to take greater ownership and control of the vertically administered national public health programmes and helping to integrate interventions for diseases with similar risks and common entry points to risk reduction.

46. Decentralizing governance and management in hospitals while ensuring participatory decision-making through representation of all categories of stakeholders in governance arrangements; allowing the incorporation of user fee only as an incentive for quality and not at the cost of creating access issues for the poor, and in such cases, using public resources to support objectives, which directly serve the equity objective.

47. Prioritizing services relevant to the poor and reorienting government services towards the disadvantaged through means that target benefits by virtue of certain characteristics or eligibility criteria.

48. Reorienting the behaviour change communication strategy to impact the behaviour of all actors in the health system; broadening the scope of health communication beyond the public service announcement approach through the use of behavioural research in areas such as persuasion and large group processes, and using social marketing as a tool to complement health reform measures.

49. Strategically using payment mechanisms and social marketing to support reform of public facilities and exploring the potential within innovative service delivery arrangements to reach the poor.

50. Improving trauma and emergency services to the extent that a credible and cost-effective analysis suggests.

7. Health Workforce

Human workforce is not just another input into the health system. They are strategic actors who can act individually or collectively to facilitate the process of health reform.

Goal: to develop a health workforce appropriate to the needs of the country's health system, giving due attention to numerical inadequacies, issues relating to mal-distribution and deployment, lack of diversity, problems with capacity building and training, and regulation; and to take into account the impact of reform in the areas of decentralization, outsourcing, granting autonomy, public-private relationships, and other areas on the health workforce and vice versa.

Strategies:

51. Developing a comprehensive human resource policy based on an objective assessment of needs. Enacting a health services law to encompass all categories of healthcare providers in order to define career structures, job descriptions, reporting relationships, and tenure policy; laying down of service, promotion, and recruitment rules after a careful assessment of health human resource needs; reviewing cadres with a view to eliminating duplication and overlap, and stipulating health provider population ratios.

52. Establishing a comprehensive and consolidated database and information system on health-related human resource in the country.

53. Addressing the current shortfall in certain categories of healthcare providers because of absolute low numbers, and in other disciplines that are high in demand and low on capacity; while doing so ensuring that efforts to enhance numbers by augmenting training are matched with appropriate retention policies and regulatory controls over

migration—both within the country outside of the state system as well as migration overseas; addressing the issue of mal-distribution, ineffective deployment, and uneven distribution through special incentives; aiming to achieve desirable healthcare provider-population ratios benchmarking international recommendations.

54. Reforming undergraduate medical education, both in terms of the content of the curriculum as well as the mode of teaching—balancing public health, health systems and health promotion with medical care and focusing on problem based learning and competency based education; improving management structures and faculty training, and revamping performance evaluation/promotion appraisals of members belonging to the teaching cadres; and enabling autonomy and de-politicization of health educational institutions.

55. Meeting the priority training needs for postgraduate education; strengthening in-service training of all categories of healthcare providers by institutionalizing professional self-development and making specified credit hours of Continuing Medical Education training a mandatory requirement for promotions as well as criteria for renewal of registration by accrediting agencies.

56. Paying due attention to staffing governance positions through merit-based hiring and appropriate deployments, and doing away with the culture of nepotism, cronyism, and patronage.

57. Using financial incentives as a tool to reform workforce behaviours in the health sector in order to address issues of staff absenteeism, dual job-holding, and lack of motivation to perform in tandem with impartial accountability and rewards for performance; paying due attention to recruitment and retention of women in the health sector workforce.

58. Exploring ways of rendering 'quacks' less harmful, and where possible, training them to contribute towards improving health outcomes.

8. Medicines and related technologies

Medicines, biopharmaceuticals and devices constitute an important input into the health system.

Goal: to make quality essential medicines and technologies, critical for the delivery of the essential health services package accessible, affordable, and consumer-friendly on an equitable basis and to promote their rational use in the health system.

Strategies:

59. Reviewing and updating the National Drug Policy 1997 and the Drug Act 1976 in order to address gaps that have emerged as a result of contemporary considerations—trends in technology and advertising and World Trade Organization agreements; reviewing and updating clauses and covenants that are exploitable with reference to product, quality, and price regulation; coordinating the medicines policy with trade, investment, intellectual property rights, and consumer protection policies; and expanding the scope of policy and legislation to cover medical devices, related healthcare technologies, health products, and traditional medicines, which are presently outside of its ambit.

60. Minimizing collusion in regulation and limiting the space for manoeuvrability by separating the functions of policy-making, implementation, and regulation in institutional arrangements; ensuring uniform implementation of policies through transparency in governance; promoting specific transparency building measures by incentivizing field regulation, adequately resourcing the drug testing infrastructure, creating windows for direct involvement of consumers, creating public awareness, and making strategic interventions to enhance distribution chain security.

61. Ensuring predictability and transparency in the pricing formula; mainstreaming measures as appropriate to rationalize costs; investing in market information systems and international price

information services and drug price indicator guides to enable procurement agencies to make evidence-based decisions; and addressing factors, which influence prescribing by health providers in the interest of access and affordability.

62. Instituting measures to check the mushrooming of spurious drugs—imposing conditional bans on the resale of machinery and restrictions on the sale of raw materials in the open market; instituting stricter penalties for violation of the law.

63. Reviewing and revising, as appropriate, procedures for drug selection, procurement, storage, dispensing, and rational prescribing and enhancing post-marketing surveillance in order to monitor and report adverse drug reactions.

64. Basing decisions on procurements, both on cost as well as quality; fostering transparency in the process of procuring and contracting through the use of technology and ensuring compliance with stated stipulations.

65. Promoting the National Essential Drug List (NEDL) as a tool for rationalizing pharmaceutical expenditure; scaling down the number of drugs, eliminating outliers in terms of usage, and updating the NEDL on a regular basis to keep it current and in line with community needs; ensuring that it is available to all the concerned stakeholders in the public and private sectors.

66. Ensuring that factors, which contribute to shortages of medicines are effectively and pragmatically addressed by allocating adequate raw material quotas, addressing genuine manufacturing bottlenecks, factoring price into consideration in order to curb smuggling of drugs habitually short in the market, countering manufacturing monopolies, stipulating multi-source registrations for medicines on the NEDL, ensuring that manufacturers maintain an uninterrupted supply of essential medicines at stable prices, and establishing an effective reporting and response mechanism to track shortages.

67. Strengthening local regulations; developing and enforcing minimum requirements in line with the international code of marketing practices to address hospitality-based incentive intense marketing practices of the commercial sector; building safeguards against conflict of interest during marketing to ensure that physicians do not get under the influence of incentives offered to them; and collaborating with medical professional bodies in order to institutionalize clinical and prescription audit.

68. Regulating the sale of medicines at private stores and mandating certified trainings for drug sellers in the private sector and the presence of pharmacists in hospital pharmacies.

69. Developing a baseline position to clearly articulate the envisaged Pakistan-specific public health impacts of WTO agreements; enhancing capacity to take advantage, as appropriate, of prerogatives that countries have, to override certain provisions of WTO in the interest of making low-cost high-quality drugs accessible to all; allocating public resources to build and support the research and development base of the national pharmaceutical industry and assisting in facilitating technology transfer to the local pharmaceutical industry, albeit with careful ethical safeguards.

70. Streamlining the already collected research and development funds from the industry for promotion of local research.

Index

E

F

O

P

Q

R

W

Y

Z